THE PART-TIME VEGETARIAN

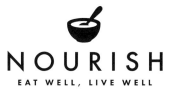

NOURISH

EAT WELL, LIVE WELL

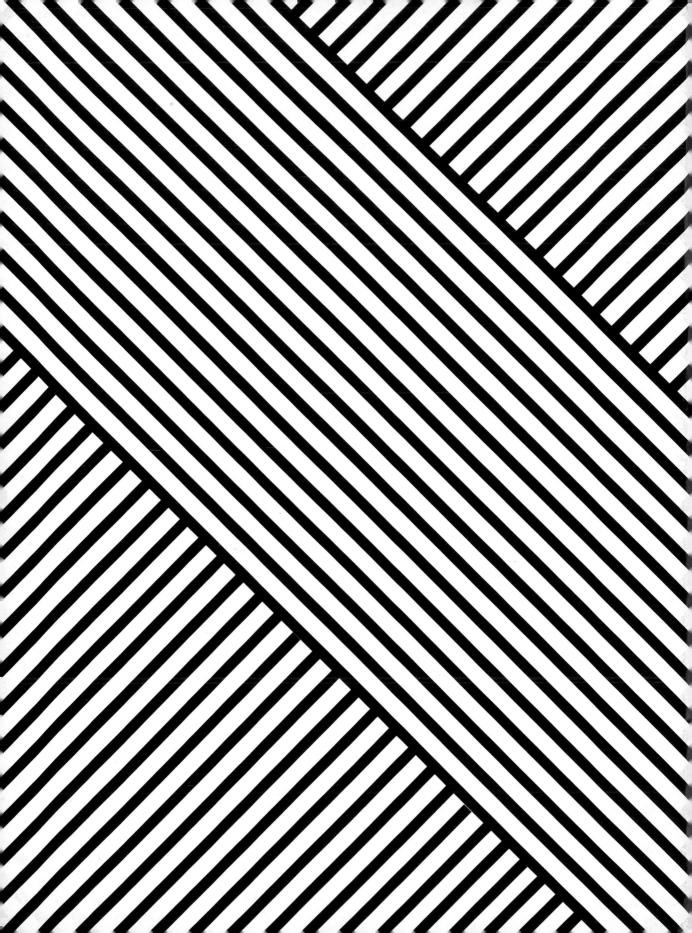

THE PART-TIME VEGETARIAN

FLEXIBLE RECIPES TO GO (NEARLY) MEAT-FREE

NICOLA GRAIMES

THE PART-TIME VEGETARIAN
Nicola Graimes

First published in the UK and USA in 2015 by Nourish,
an imprint of Watkins Media Limited
19 Cecil Court
London WC2N 4EZ

enquiries@nourishbooks.com

Publisher: Grace Cheetham
Managing Editor: Rebecca Woods
Editor: Wendy Hobson
Managing Designer: Georgina Hewitt
Designer: Allan Sommerville
Commissioned photography: Haarala Hamilton
Food Stylist: Sara Lewis
Prop Stylist: Haarala Hamilton
Production: Uzma Taj

A CIP record for this book is available from the British Library

ISBN: 978-1-84899-265-8

10 9 8 7 6 5 4

Typeset in Gill Sans
Colour reproduction by XY Digital
Printed in China

Notes on the Recipes
Unless otherwise stated:
– Use medium eggs, fruit and vegetables
– Use fresh ingredients, including herbs and spices
– Do not mix metric and imperial measurements
– 1 tsp = 5ml   1 tbsp = 15ml   1 cup = 240ml

Publisher's Note
While every care has been taken in compiling the recipes for this book,
Watkins Media Limited, or any other persons who have been involved in
working on this publication, cannot accept responsibility for any errors or
omissions, inadvertent or not, that may be found in the recipes or text, nor
for any problems that may arise as a result of preparing one of these recipes.
If you are pregnant or breastfeeding or have any special dietary requirements
or medical conditions, it is advisable to consult a medical professional before
following any of the recipes contained in this book.

nourishbooks.com

CONTENTS

Introduction

It's time to make a confession: writing this book is a bit of a coming out for me. Having been vegetarian for nearly thirty years, I've started including a small amount of meat and fish in my diet. This change of heart – and eating habits – has come about due to various reasons and really wasn't taken lightly. Yet I've discovered that I'm not alone as the number of what I suppose could be called 'part-time vegetarians' is growing exponentially on a yearly basis. A study by the *American Journal of Clinical Nutrition* found that nearly two out of three 'vegetarians' occasionally like to eat meat, chicken or fish.

There is also a significant rise in the number of non-vegetarians who eat meat-free meals on a regular basis. Until relatively recently, many non-vegetarians would have scoffed at the idea of deliberately choosing to eat vegetable-based meals several times a week, but there has been an impressive positive shift in many of our eating habits and part of this is cutting down on the amount of meat we eat.

It's fantastic that many of us are becoming more conscious of what we eat and where our food comes from. It's all a bit clichéd, but vegetarian food has come a long way since the lentil days – not that there is anything wrong with lentils! But while in the past it may have sometimes been seen as a little too worthy, vegetarian cooking is now exciting, inventive and inspirational. There has been an explosion of different ingredients available from all corners of the globe, while many restaurants – not just vegetarian ones – and numerous cookery writers and food bloggers have fuelled the growing interest in what they are calling 'flexitarianism' or flexible eating.

COMMON FACTORS

So what is a flexitarian diet and why should we be interested?

Just like vegetarians, part-time vegetarians – or flexitarians – prefer to base meals on vegetables. Whether this is for health, economic or moral reasons (or more likely a combination of all three), the fact is that the flexitarian diet – one that is largely vegetarian, but occasionally includes poultry, meat and seafood – is growing in popularity and is a long-term trend that's gaining momentum.

Since we have all become more thrifty and price-conscious when food shopping, and vegetables on the whole are a lot cheaper than meat and fish, the part-time vegetarian diet seems to be the logical way to go for non-vegetarians. Good-quality meat and fish have become prohibitively expensive, so it makes sense to eat them less often so you can still choose the best quality and ethically sourced.

In the eyes of food scientists, our current consumption of meat and fish cannot be sustained in the long-term. It is far more ecologically sound to eat more vegetables, which are much less intrusive on the earth's resources than meat products.

What's more, the numerous health benefits of a vegetarian diet are well documented and have become more poignant due to various health scares that have blighted some areas of food production in recent years. All these factors mark a shift towards a vegetable-based diet or a meat-light one.

As the name suggests, the beauty of this diet is its flexibility. Unlike most diets it's not prescriptive – there are no hard-and-fast rules – so it can easily be adapted to suit your lifestyle and what's happening on a weekly basis. Whether you opt to go meat-free just one day a week, eat meat on rare occasions or prefer to choose meat- and fish-light meals, *The Part-time Vegetarian* allows you that flexibility. The book is also perfect for those who are fully fledged vegetarians, or who have a non-meat eater in the family or coming for dinner, and are looking for new ideas and adaptable recipes that don't rely on meat substitutes.

In other words, *The Part-time Vegetarian* cookbook is for those looking for simple, nourishing, cost-effective meals and an environmentally intelligent way to eat. Flexitarians are taking a positive step forward when it comes to their health, the environment and animals.

WHY GO FLEXITARIAN?

There are many motivations for going flexitarian. The ultimate goal may or may not be to become vegetarian or vegan in time, but there are lots of reasons to make positive changes to your diet by reducing the amount of meat you eat.

❭ **HEALTH:** numerous studies point to the positive health benefits of a plant-based diet, particularly in reducing the risk of chronic illnesses such as heart disease, certain types of cancer, high blood pressure and obesity.

❭ **ANIMAL WELFARE:** scandals relating to the farming of animals and processing has made us nervous and suspicious of what we're actually buying. As well as cutting back on meat, a positive

change flexitarians can make is to look for meat that has been ethically reared to a high standard of animal welfare. Choose free-range, organic and locally reared, if possible, and give a plant-based diet greater priority.

❭ **ENVIRONMENT:** studies estimate that an affluent diet containing significant amounts of meat requires up to three times as many resources as a vegetarian diet. One of the simplest changes we can make is to buy locally and eat seasonally. If produced locally, food has less impact on the environment, thanks to reduced energy use and associated CO_2 emissions. Buying seasonal fruit and vegetables is also a good way to support the local economy and farming communities.

About this book

Vegetarian food has moved on… It has progressed in inspirational leaps and bounds away from stodgy, worthy and dairy-laden dishes to bright, fresh, interesting meals full of flavour, texture and colour. There's been a real shift in enthusiasm for meat-free cooking and a growing willingness by cooks to experiment with new ways of preparing and presenting vegetables and other vegetarian ingredients. It wasn't long ago that many top-name chefs would openly dismiss vegetarian food as unworthy of recognition – how things change.

Consequently, *The Part-time Vegetarian* is a celebration of vegetarian food with well over 120 simple and nourishing recipes that take you from Breakfasts and Brunches; Light Meals, ideal for lunches or snacks; quick and easy Weekday Suppers; Weekend Cooking for when time is not so pressing; to Food for Sharing, covering dishes for entertaining, celebrations and special occasions.

But there's more…. perhaps refreshingly, our eating habits are not often easy to pigeonhole, so the idea behind *The Part-time Vegetarian* was born out of the growing trend in flexitarianism, primarily a plant-based diet with the occasional addition of meat or seafood. In keeping with those who do not want to commit to a fully vegetarian diet, choosing a more flexible way of eating instead, many of the recipes in this book can readily be adapted to include meat, poultry or seafood. However, rather than taking centre stage, they are not the main focus of the recipes, which value the impressive range of vegetables, grains, legumes, nuts, eggs and dairy foods instead.

In the book, you'll find that many of the vegetarian recipes have a 'Part-time Variation' at the end, a twist that means you have effectively two recipes in one. Sometimes the variation is as simple as a token sprinkling of crispy bacon on the finished dish, at other times it's a more substantial addition. Though having said that, the recipes remain intentionally meat- or seafood-light throughout. The Part-time Variations add a new dimension to the vegetarian recipes and consequently widen and extend the home cook's repertoire of dishes. For instance, the Udon Noodle Broth (see page 59) can easily be adapted with the addition of prawns/shrimp. Alternatively, instead of the roasted mushrooms served on a white bean mash (see page 105), there is spiced grilled lamb. A change in the main ingredient sometimes calls for a slight switch in spicing or use of other flavourings, and it is these minor alterations that can take a dish and turn it into something quite different.

All the recipes are inherently easy to make but may differ, if that's not a contradiction, in their complexity and the length of time they take to make – so there's something for everyone, from the new cook to the more accomplished one. Likewise, there are ideas for quick and easy breakfasts, brunches, snacks, lunches and weekday suppers. But for days when time is not so pressing – if that's ever possible – or you are looking to make a dish for a special occasion, then you'll find recipes to suit. Also, where a recipe calls for a slightly more unusual or unfamiliar ingredient, I've been mindful to give an alternative just in case.

Additionally, within each chapter, you'll find a special feature comprising simple, pocket-size recipes that have been chosen to enhance or complement the flexible recipes in the book. This eclectic bunch includes Spreads, Butters and Ketchups; Chutneys, Dips and Salsas; Dressings; Pickles and Ferments; and Sauces. Some of the feature recipes form an essential part of a main recipe, while others make an interesting side dish or add extra pizzazz.

Whether it's an intricate celebratory pie or a five-minute fresh relish, at the heart of *The Part-time Vegetarian* is a desire to entice those who wish to increase their repertoire of meat-free meals, whether cooking for themselves or family and friends. Most importantly, the book appreciates and celebrates the diversity of a flexitarian way of eating.

WHERE TO START...

If you are contemplating cutting down on meat on your way to becoming a full-time vegetarian or have reintroduced meat and seafood into your diet, the following pointers may help.

⟩ **Choose sustainable fish:** on the surface, fish meets all the demands of a healthy lifestyle: it's nutritious, versatile and quick, but a decline in fish stocks means that it has become essential to buy sustainably. Look for the blue MSC (Marine Stewardship Council) label, which certifies good fishing practices, protects marine life and helps support fishing communities. It pays to be fish aware, so check out: fish that is in season and not in danger; responsibly farmed fish; river fish; and if you're lucky enough to live near the coast, local fish schemes.

⟩ **Opt for free-range and organic:** provenance is becoming an important priority so whenever feasible and economics allow, buy ethically reared meat and poultry. Make the most of economical cuts of meat, which are perfect for slow-cooked stews and roasts. Leftover roasted meats can be transformed into a second meal, while the bones are the perfect base for a good homemade stock.

⟩ **Be aware of seasonality:** it's not only fresh produce that is seasonal, certain meat and seafoods are influenced by the seasons, too. If available, try to buy locally produced food. Not only will you be cutting down on the food miles your shopping has travelled and supporting the local community, the produce is likely to be fresher.

⟩ **Eat up your veg:** make vegetables the main focus of every meal. Buying locally can be a good way of keeping costs down and supporting the local economy, while local markets and box delivery schemes ensure you get seasonal produce. The meal plans at the back of the book (pages 216–219) will give you plenty of ideas for different ways to use veg.

The part-time vegetarian kitchen

These are a few of my favourite things… or so go the lyrics to the famous song! This eclectic list of predominantly store cupboard ingredients crop up throughout *The Part-time Vegetarian* and while some may be new to you, others will be more than familiar but are still worth a mention. In places, alternatives are given for the more unusual or hard-to-find ingredients. The following list is presented by type of ingredient as well as alphabetical order for easy reference.

VEGETABLES

It's only right that vegetables come top of the list, for they are at the heart of this book. We have a new love for vegetables, but it's easy to get stuck in a rut when it comes to buying fresh produce, settling for pretty much the same every week. There's nothing wrong with having favourite veg, but it's worth opening your eyes to new varieties that aren't on the regulars list. Kolhrabi, turnip, cauliflower, kale, hispi cabbage, pak choi/bok choy, broad/fava beans and celeriac/celery root are new-found or revived favourites. Seasonal veg is always best, if possible, and frozen is a good – or sometimes even better – option (see page 15).

HERBS & SPICES

⊃ **CARDAMOM:** a favourite spice, the whole pods can either be split or lightly crushed and added to Middle Eastern and Asian curries, soups and stews, to the cooking water for rice and other grains and, perhaps surprisingly, to Scandinavian baked goods. For a more intense spicy-sweet flavour, roast and grind the seeds to give an aromatic warmth to sweet and savoury dishes.

⊃ **CHIPOTLE CHILLI:** you get a lot of bang for your buck with the chipotle in terms of flavour. This smoked dried jalapeño comes in powder, paste and dried whole form and adds a distinctive heat and smokiness to Mexican and Tex-Mex cooking, and is especially good in bean and grain dishes. The dried chilli needs rehydrating in hot water.

⊃ **CORIANDER SEEDS:** known for their earthy, mildly lemony flavour, coriander seeds feature alongside cumin as a key spice in Indian curries and Middle Eastern dishes, and are also a popular pickling spice. For the best flavour, toast the seeds in a dry frying pan for a minute or so until they start to smell aromatic, then leave to cool and either use whole or grind to a powder.

⊃ **DRIED HERBS:** although I prefer to use fresh, there is a place for certain dried herbs in the store cupboard, particularly during the winter months. Oregano, thyme, marjoram and, to a lesser extent, mint (although the dried version is good sprinkled over some Middle Eastern and Mediterranean salads and grain dishes) all dry well.

⊃ **HARISSA:** most usually a mix of chilli, garlic, coriander, cumin, smoked paprika, mint and tomato, harissa comes in powder and paste form and is perfect for enlivening couscous, stews, sauces and marinades. Look out for rose harissa with its addition of rose petals, which lend a wonderful fragrant twist. For an easy marinade, simply stir a spoonful of the North African and Middle Eastern herb and spice mix into olive oil and spread over a mixture of aubergine/eggplant, sweet peppers, courgettes/zucchini, onions and sweet potatoes before roasting to add a fragrant chilli heat and crust.

⊃ **NIGELLA SEEDS:** a few of these nutty, slightly bitter, tiny black seeds (also known as black onion seeds) go a long way. I like to sprinkle them over flatbreads and salads and into rice, pilafs and curries to add a quick flavour boost.

⊃ **SMOKED PAPRIKA:** the flavour of Spanish smoked paprika is unmistakeable. With its rich, oaky, smokiness, the paprika ranges in heat from sweet and mild to picante or hot and lends heaps of flavour as well as colour to marinades, stews, soups and dressings. Look out for the authentic Spanish, *pimentón de la vera*.

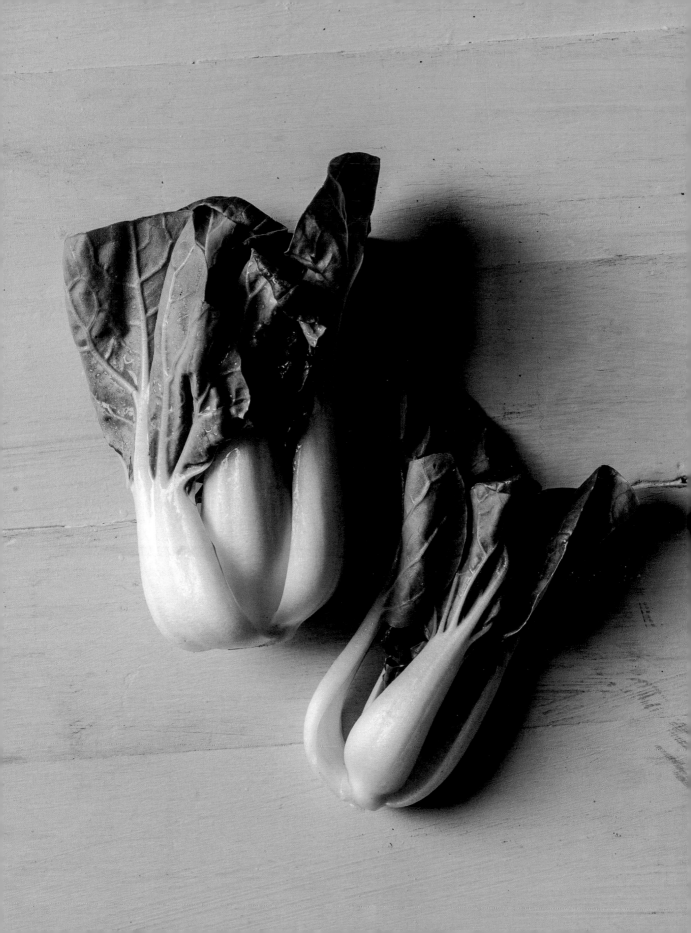

▹ **STAR ANISE:** with its attractive star shape and distinctive warm, liquorice notes, the spice is central to Chinese cooking. Use it in aromatic Asian curries, stir-fries, broths and hotpots as well as a flavouring for sweet custards and fruit compôtes.

▹ **SUMAC:** at one time this reddish-brown spice was only available in Middle Eastern shops, but thanks to the increased popularity of cooking from this part of the world – the Ottolenghi factor – you can now find it in many large supermarkets. The ground, dried berries with their astringent, sour flavour are a key ingredient in *dukkah* (see page 67), the Egyptian seed, spice and nut mix.

▹ **TAMARIND:** buy this sweet-sour fruit in a compressed block of pulp or as a paste. Originally the pulp of a long, bean-like pod, the block is closer in flavour to the original fruit than the jars of paste you can buy, but you'll have to soak it first to soften it to its puréed-date texture as well as pick out the large seeds. Use tamarind to add a sour note to chutneys, curries and marinades.

▹ **TOGARASHI:** a sprinkling of this Japanese spice blend (also known as *shichimi togarashi*) adds a lively citrus-chilli lift to noodle and rice dishes, salads, dressings and marinades. Like the spice mix harissa, there are many versions available, but a combination of chilli, orange peel, sansho, sesame seeds and nori is most common. You can make your own blend or buy ready-made in Asian grocers or large supermarkets.

SAUCES & CONDIMENTS

▹ **CHINESE RICE WINE:** second only in importance to soy sauce in Chinese cooking, this sweet wine can be swapped with dry sherry if you find it difficult to get hold of.

▹ **KECAP MANIS:** this Indonesian sweet soy sauce is almost syrupy in consistency and adds a sticky, spicy sweetness to marinades, dressings and dips. It is possible to make your own version by combining 3 tablespoons dark soy sauce with 1 heaped teaspoon soft brown sugar and a pinch of ground star anise.

▹ **MIRIN:** a splash of this slightly syrupy sweetened rice wine in a marinade adds a glossy glaze to grilled, roasted and stir-fried foods. If you can't find it, dry sherry makes a worthy alternative, as does Chinese rice wine or slightly sweet white wine – or maybe that's sacrilege.

▹ **MISO PASTE:** a spoonful of this intense fermented soya, barley, wheat or rice paste makes a simple restorative broth, but its uses are far wider. Don't limit miso to oriental dishes – marinades, dressings, stews and sauces all benefit from its savoury umami quality, which varies in depth of flavour depending on its colour – brown, red, yellow and white. Generally, the darker the colour, the stronger the flavour of the paste. A jar of miso will keep for weeks stored in the refrigerator.

▹ **RICE VINEGAR:** generally less acidic than wine vinegar, there are many types of rice vinegar. Ideal for pickling ginger and vegetables when you don't want the finished result to be too harsh, rice vinegar ranges from the slightly sweeter Japanese to the sharper Chinese versions that vary in colour from pale to deep red and black. There are no true Western alternatives, but if push comes to shove use a good-quality white wine vinegar slightly sweetened with caster/granulated sugar, or you could use balsamic vinegar instead of Chinese black vinegar.

▹ **TAHINI:** a jar of this rich, thick sesame seed paste is a must in my kitchen. Not only does it add a deep, nutty flavour to both Middle Eastern and Japanese dishes, it's an easy way to add a protein-rich, nutritious boost to anything from stews and noodle broths to dressings and sauces. It's also indispensable in humous and the aubergine/eggplant purée, *baba ganoush*. For a quick dressing, mix together tahini, plain yogurt, crushed garlic, lemon juice and seasoning and loosen it with a little hot water if too thick. The light-coloured tahini is preferred as it is not as bitter as the darker alternative.

⟩ **YUZU:** find this intensely flavoured, vibrant yellow juice in small bottles in the condiments or Asian sections in large supermarkets or Asian grocers. The juice comes from the yuzu fruit, which looks like a knobbly mandarin and has a flavour that could best be described as a cross between a lemon and a grapefruit. Popular in Japanese cooking for its intense citrus taste, you could replace the juice with other citrus fruit such as lemon, lime or white-fleshed grapefruit.

OILS

⟩ **COCONUT OIL:** this pure white solid fat, which liquifies when heated, has become **the** oil of the moment. It's highly stable, so that means it can happily be heated to high temperatures, is less prone to rancidity than most other oils and has many impressive reputed health benefits. For cooking, look for extra virgin or organic coconut oil as they are less likely to be chemically processed and are therefore purer, retaining their health properties. For me, coconut oil works best in Asian curries, stir-fries and pilaus as well as North African tagines, pilafs and similar. A big bonus is that the oil makes an excellent moisturiser and hair conditioner.

⟩ **RAPESEED/CANOLA OIL (cold pressed):** while it goes without saying that a good-quality extra virgin olive oil is a 'must-have' in the kitchen, cold-pressed rapeseed/canola oil has impressive credentials. Along with its inviting vibrant colour that lends a golden hue to whatever you're cooking, it's a highly stable oil when heated with a high smoking point. Therefore it suits use in stir-fries as well as marinades, griddled/grilled foods, roasts and salad dressings, although it would be pretty wasteful to use a high-end rapeseed/canola oil for deep frying. It's important to look for an unblended cold-pressed oil, which is extracted from the seed without the use of chemicals and retains its numerous health benefits. Its mild flavour also lends itself to home-made mayonnaise or aioli, when a more dominant olive oil can overpower or be too bitter.

GRAINS & BEANS

⟩ **BLACK RICE:** striking in salads when combined with contrasting ingredients, this good-looking, medium-grain rice keeps its shape when cooked and has a lovely nutty flavour and texture. Brown basmati makes a suitable, if perhaps slightly less dramatic, alternative.

⟩ **GRAM FLOUR:** also known as chickpea or besan, this pale yellow flour is a staple in Asian cooking where it's used use to make batter for pakoras as well as flatbreads and fritters. Perhaps surprisingly, the distinctively flavoured, slightly earthy-tasting flour is well travelled since it is also used to make *farinata*, a type of thick pancake in northern Italy and *socca*, a similar version in the south of France.

⟩ **FREEKEH:** though this green unripe wheat is new to most of us, it's been around for hundreds of years and makes a delicious alternative to rice (but with extra substance) and other grains in pilafs and salads, or as an accompaniment. What makes the grain different to most others is its slightly smoky, nutty flavour, which comes from being roasted over wood fires.

⟩ **KAMUT:** the trademarked name for the ancient type of wheat known as *khorasan,* this rediscovered grain is now grown in North America as well as the Middle East. It is an attractive golden-coloured grain that keeps its shape after cooking. Although the grain contains gluten, many who find they are intolerant to modern strains of wheat can eat protein-rich Kamut. Find the grain in health food shops and large supermarkets. Barley makes a good alternative.

◐ **POLENTA:** the beauty of this fine yellow cornmeal is its versatility. It makes a welcome change from other types of carbs, particularly as an alternative to mashed potatoes or chips, as a base for bruschetta and pizzas, or as a pie crust. There's something very pleasing about stirring a spluttering pot of polenta and, while it makes the perfect comfort food served plain with a knob of butter, try adding other flavours, such as a good handful of grated Parmesan or other cheese, flavoured oils, pesto, herbs, chilli and other spices. I've even added Thai flavours with delicious results.

◐ **PUY LENTILS:** I'm a big fan of lentils of all types (and beans for that matter). Puy not only have an attractive marbled blue-green colour, they retain their shape after cooking, so add substance and nutritional value to salads, hotpots and soups. Unlike dried beans, lentils don't require pre-soaking and are much quicker to cook, but for super-quick lentils, you can't beat canned ones that just need heating through. For a quick, warming lunch, sauté mushrooms, garlic, tomato and kale and stir in cooked Puy lentils, hot smoked paprika and thyme. A squeeze of lemon juice and seasoning adds the finishing touch. This works equally well with canned chickpeas, butter beans and cannellini beans, too.

◐ **QUINOA:** hailed as a 'super-grain', the tiny, bead-like seeds make a protein-rich alternative to grains such as couscous and bulghur wheat. Look out for the distinctive, nutty red and black quinoas, along with the more usual neutral-coloured one. With its mild, slightly bitter flavour, it benefits from combining with spices and herbs or as part of a salad. Flaked quinoa, too, is excellent in muesli and porridge/oatmeal.

AND MORE...

◐ **CAPERS:** it's taken a while for me to get into capers, but a turning point was discovering the small, peppercorn-sized, strangely named *nonpareil*, which are absolutely

delicious fried in olive oil until crisp. The salty, briny berries are also great finely chopped into a salsa verde, tapenade, salsa, pesto or relish, or any type of buttery sauce when you want to add a touch of acidity.

◐ **CHESTNUTS:** nothing quite matches the smell of roasting chestnuts, yet a vacuum pack of ready-cooked and peeled ones makes a useful and convenient store cupboard standby. Chestnuts add a rich, earthy, 'meaty' substance to casseroles and can be mashed into stuffings and vegetable roasts or puréed into pâtés.

◐ **SEA VEGETABLES:** the West has been relatively slow to catch on to seaweed, but thanks to the growing popularity of sushi we've become more open to using it in cooking and appreciating its impressive health benefits. Sushi lovers will be familiar with nori sheets, but you can also find nori flakes or make your own: simply use tongs to hold a sheet of nori over a hob/stovetop for a minute, moving it so it toasts evenly and turns crisp. Leave to cool then crumble over noodle salads, stir-fries and broths.

Other favourite sea vegetables are dulse and wakame. The former has purple-brown flat fronds with a mildly spicy flavour when soaked from dried, but can also be toasted or dry-fried when it takes on a salty, slightly 'bacon' flavour. Wakame, on the other hand, has a definite hint of the sea in flavour and delicate green fronds when rehydrated.

◐ **SEEDS:** they may look small and unassuming but seeds – sesame, sunflower, pumpkin and hemp – are nutritious and versatile. A daily part of my diet, whether added to breakfast muesli, toasted and sprinkled over stir-fries, as a nutty crunch in salads and pilafs, or ground into pastes and dips, they are indispensable. This is perhaps more true of sesame seeds than any other, as the tiny cream-coloured seeds are a fundamental part of the Middle Eastern spice condiments, *dukkah* and *za'atar*, as well as the creamy paste, tahini – a must in humous.

TOFU (& TEMPEH): you either love it or hate it… and I'm in the former camp. Rather than seeing it as bland, I like to think of it as a blank canvas, a vehicle for flavouring with all manner of herbs, spices and marinades – and not just Asian flavours. The methods of cooking tofu, or soya beancurd, are equally versatile: roast, stir-fried, grilled, griddled or smoked, they all lend a different quality to the protein-rich ingredient. Likewise, tempeh can be used in similar ways to tofu. Made by fermenting soya beans with a cultured starter, tempeh has a firmer, denser texture than tofu with a nutty, savoury flavour.

FREEZER

A full freezer costs less to run than a half-empty one, so it's worth making the most of this invaluable storage space. It pays to be organized, labelling foods and dating them before freezing, especially if you, like me, have a tendency to fill your freezer with pots of leftover wine (for use in sauces, risottos, gravies and stews); bread (some processed into crumbs); foraged berries and other fruit; surplus egg whites; homemade stock and various meals made in bulk. There are also a few shop-bought must-haves, including:

VEGETABLES: some vegetables take to freezing better than others. If you regularly find yourself throwing away bags of fresh spinach that are past their best, then frozen leaf spinach is indispensable. Avoid the chopped spinach, which is prone to turn to mush when cooked, and go for leaf spinach instead and, since it is usually frozen in handy individual portions, it's super convenient.

The short growing season of fresh peas as well as broad/fava beans, makes them both an obvious choice for the freezer. Frozen peas are a godsend: the small petit pois are sweet and tender, while the more economical garden peas are perfect blended into soups, mashed with cooked potato or can be transformed into fritters. Broad/fava beans are best popped out of their grey outer shell after cooking to reveal bright green, succulent beans inside.

A bag of endamame beans (fresh soya beans), now readily available from large supermarkets and Asian grocers, also makes a useful addition to the freezer, and the beans can be added to oriental broths, stir-fries, noodle dishes or mashed into fritters and croquettes.

LIME LEAVES & LEMONGRASS: if you find a good source of fresh kaffir lime leaves, sticks of lemongrass and fresh curry leaves, it pays to buy them in bulk – what's more they all freeze well. Open freeze on a baking sheet, then transfer to an airtight container or zip-lock freezer bag and return them to the freezer – there's no need to defrost them before use.

HERBS: certain fresh herbs freeze better than others and not surprisingly the more sturdy varieties, such as sage, rosemary, thyme and bay leaves fare much better than more delicate leaves. You can also freeze fresh parsley, chives and coriander/cilantro, but once frozen they are best used in cooked dishes. Freeze herbs laid out on a baking sheet, then transfer to a zip-lock freezer bag once frozen.

WONTON WRAPPERS: there are a few recipes in this book that use wonton wrappers. The thin pastry squares or rounds can usually be found in Chinese grocers in the freezer (or sometimes chiller) cabinet. They come stacked in packets and you simply need to defrost and peel them off one by one to use. When using, keep them covered to prevent drying out, and then the ones you don't use can be refrozen. There tends to be two types: slightly thinner for frying and thicker ones for steaming.

PUFF PASTRY: last but not least, few people now have the time or the inclination to make their own puff pastry and a pack of either the ready-rolled or a block (the latter is more economical) in the freezer is a must-have. Frozen puff takes little time to defrost and can be transformed into delicious sweet and savoury tarts, pies and tartines in next to no time.

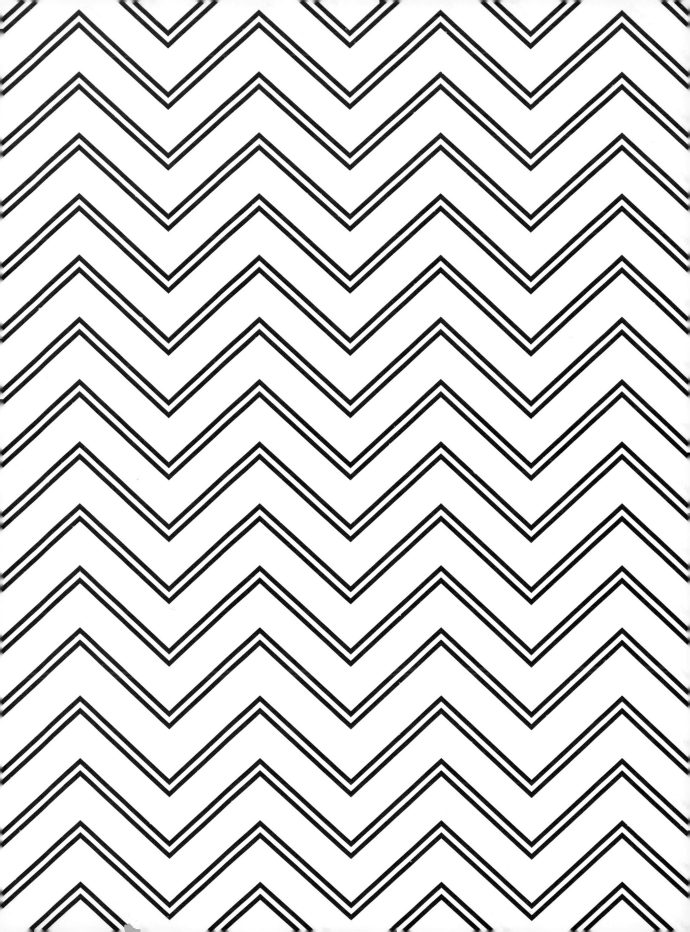

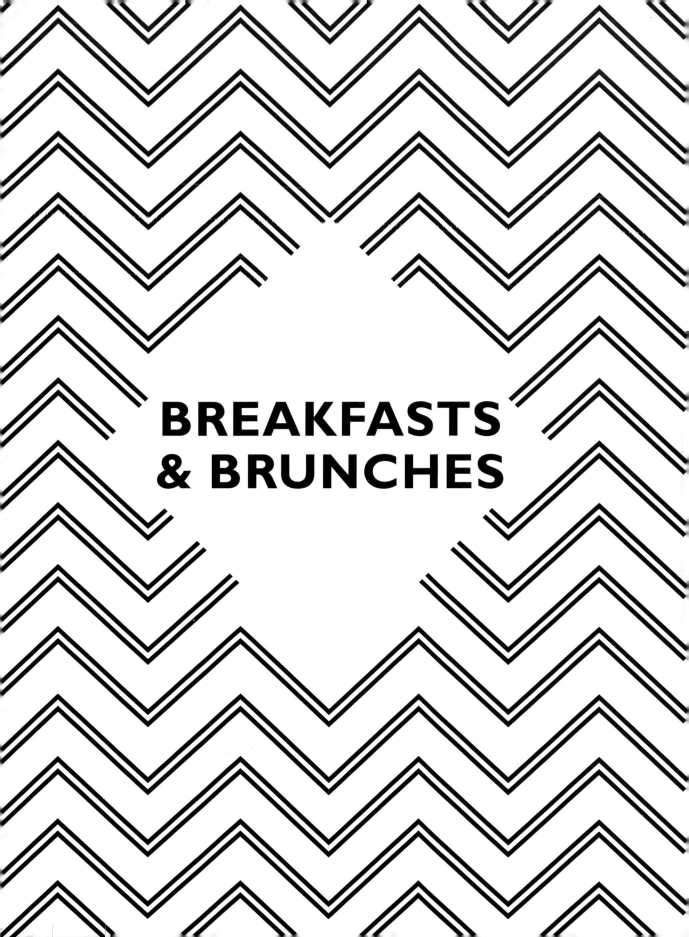

BREAKFASTS
& BRUNCHES

Nut butter AND cinnamon smoothie

SERVES ⟩⟩⟩ **2–3**

Preparation time ⟩ 5 minutes

200ml/7fl oz/scant 1 cup dairy or
non-dairy milk

4 tbsp thick plain yogurt

½ tsp ground cinnamon, plus extra
for sprinkling

2 bananas, sliced

2 tbsp Almond and Cashew Butter
(see page 41)

Both nourishing and sustaining, this creamy smoothie will help set you up for the morning ahead. You'll have some of the home-made almond and cashew nut butter left, so transfer any leftovers to a screw-topped jar and keep it in the refrigerator for up to 2 weeks – below you'll find some savoury vegetarian and non-veggie suggestions on ways to use it.

⟩⟩⟩ Put the milk, yogurt, cinnamon, bananas and Almond and Cashew Butter in a blender and blend until smooth and creamy.

⟩⟩⟩ Pour into glasses and serve with a sprinkling of cinnamon.

PART-TIME VARIATIONS

⟩⟩⟩ Vegetable, chicken or seafood satay

Use the nut butter as the base for a satay sauce to go with grilled/broiled or roasted vegetables, chicken and seafood or noodle dishes. Simply mix together 4 tbsp nut butter with 1 tbsp each of light soy sauce, hoisin sauce and sesame oil. Stir in 1 tsp jaggery, soft brown sugar or honey, 1 crushed garlic clove, 4 tbsp coconut milk, the juice of ½ lime and ½ finely chopped red chilli.

⟩⟩⟩ Malaysian-style chicken curry

To make a curry for 4 people, heat together 400g/14oz can coconut milk, 200ml/7fl oz/scant 1 cup chicken stock and 6 tbsp of the nut butter. Stir in 2 tbsp light soy sauce, 1 tbsp medium curry powder, 1 tsp dried chilli/hot pepper flakes and 1 tsp turmeric. Add 450g/1lb sliced skinless, boneless chicken breast to the sauce and cook for 5–8 minutes, adding a splash more water or stock, if the sauce is too dry. Serve with sticky rice or noodles. You could add prawns/shrimp and/or vegetables to the sauce.

⟩⟩⟩ Mung bean and nut butter humous

Stir 2 tbsp of the nut butter into the Mung Bean Humous (see page 71).

What's-in-the-cupboard muesli

I'm a creature of habit and this is pretty much my regular daily breakfast – bar the occasional bowl of porridge or granola. To avoid boredom and complacency, however, I do like to vary the fresh fruit and mix up the blend of grains, nuts and seeds. The day seems almost incomplete without this daily ritual.

》》》 Put the oats in a bowl with the flaxseeds, hemp seeds, if using, nuts, seeds, dried fruit and fresh fruit. Pour over enough milk to cover and add a few spoonfuls of yogurt, if you like.

》》》 You could make a large batch of the grain, nut, seed and dried fruit mixture, then store it in an airtight container for up to 2 weeks.

PART-TIME VARIATION

》》》 Orange bircher muesli

Soak 2 good handfuls of jumbo oats in 150ml/5fl oz/scant ⅔ cup freshly squeezed orange juice. Leave to soak for at least 1 hour or overnight, then stir in 1 tbsp ground flaxseeds and/or 1 tbsp hulled hemp seeds, 2 roughly chopped Brazil nuts, 6 broken walnut halves, 2 tbsp sunflower seeds, 1 tbsp pumpkin seeds and 3 dried dates. Stir in 2 tsp raw cacao nibs, if you like, and a good pinch each of ground cinnamon and finely grated orange zest. Pour over enough almond or oat milk to cover and serve.

SERVES 》》》 1
Preparation time ⟩ 10 minutes

2 handfuls of jumbo oats or flaked
    quinoa, barley or millet
1 tbsp ground flaxseeds and/or hulled
    hemp seeds
2 large Brazil nuts, roughly chopped
6 walnut halves, broken
2 tbsp sunflower seeds
1 tbsp pumpkin seeds
3 dried dates, apricots, figs or
    a handful of raisins
1 apple or pear, cored and grated,
    or a handful of strawberries or
    raspberries or other favourite fruit
almond milk or other dairy-free milk
    and/or plain yogurt, to serve

Quinoa granola

MAKES ⟩⟩⟩ **ABOUT 10 SERVINGS**

Preparation time ⟩ 15 minutes
Cooking time ⟩ 30 minutes

150g/5½oz/1½ cups flaked quinoa
135g/4¾oz/1½ cups jumbo oats
85g/3oz/heaped ½ cup sunflower
    seeds
85g/3oz/heaped ½ cup pumpkin seeds
100g/3½oz/¾ cup blanched almonds
100g/3½oz/1 cup pecan halves
2 tsp ground cinnamon
80ml/2½fl oz/⅓ cup coconut oil
5 tbsp clear honey
1 tsp vanilla extract
50g/1¾oz/⅓ cup dried apricots,
    roughly chopped
50g/1¾oz/⅓ cup unsweetened dried
    sour cherries, roughly chopped
raspberries, blueberries and plain
    yogurt or milk, to serve

Granola can be expensive to buy and often disappoints, being overly sugary or lacking in variety. This nutritious combination of nuts, seeds, grains and dried fruit is a favourite blend, but feel free to adapt it to use your preferred ingredients. Flaked quinoa can be found in health food shops, but if you have trouble tracking it down, increase the quantity of oats, or you could try barley or millet flakes.

⟩⟩⟩ Preheat the oven to 170°C/325°F/Gas 3. Put the quinoa, oats, seeds, nuts and cinnamon in a large mixing bowl and stir until combined.

⟩⟩⟩ Heat the coconut oil and honey in a small pan, stirring occasionally, until melted and warmed through. Remove from the heat and stir in the vanilla.

⟩⟩⟩ Pour the coconut oil mixture over the dry ingredients in the bowl and stir until everything is mixed together well.

⟩⟩⟩ Tip the granola mixture onto two large baking sheets and spread it out into an even layer. Bake for 30 minutes, turning once, until slightly golden and crisp. Transfer the granola to the mixing bowl and stir in the apricots and cherries. Leave to cool.

⟩⟩⟩ Serve the granola with raspberries, blueberries and yogurt or milk. Store any remaining granola in an airtight jar for up to 2 weeks.

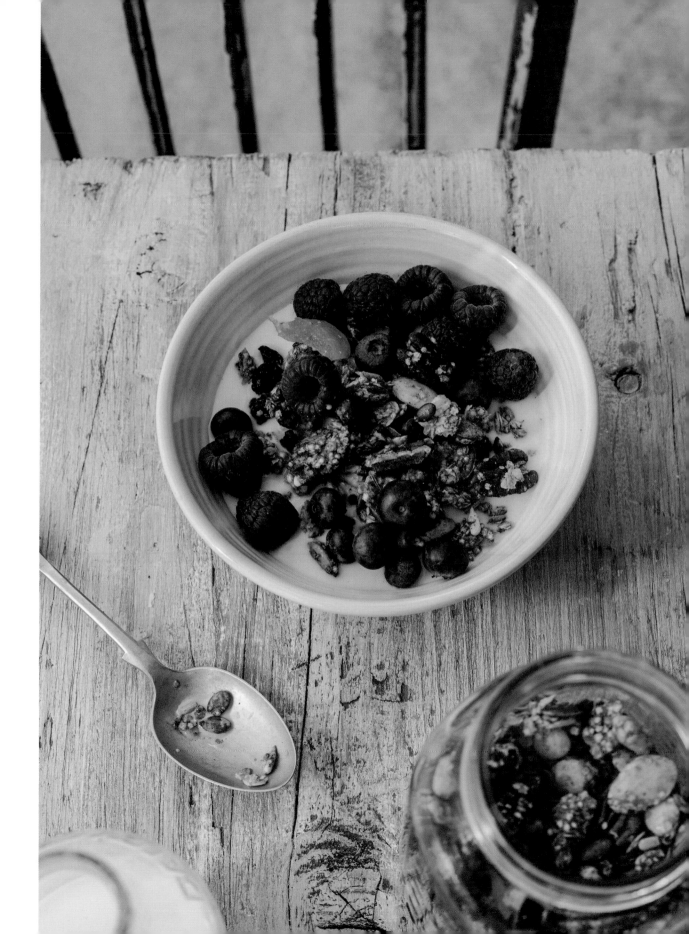

Savoury miso porridge
WITH cashews

SERVES ⟫⟫ **3–4**

Preparation time ⟩ 10 minutes
Cooking time ⟩ 20 minutes

2 handfuls of cashew nuts
1 tbsp butter
2 eggs, lightly beaten
200g/7oz/heaped 2 cups jumbo
    rolled oats
2.5cm/1in piece of fresh root ginger,
    peeled and finely chopped
4 tbsp brown rice miso paste
2 tbsp light soy sauce
nori flakes, for sprinkling (optional)

To be honest, I wasn't sure that the concept of a savoury porridge was going to work, but I was pleasantly surprised – it's simply a hug in a bowl. The premise is a Western twist on the typical Japanese breakfast of steamed rice, miso soup, and various accompaniments. For a touch of authenticity, serve the savoury, omelette-topped porridge with small bowls of natto (fermented soy beans) and Japanese pickles, such as umeboshi plums, on the side.

⟫⟫ Toast the cashews in a dry non-stick frying pan over a medium heat for 5 minutes, turning once, until starting to colour. Remove from the pan, roughly chop and leave to one side.

⟫⟫ To make the omelette, melt the butter in the pan. Pour in the eggs, tilting the pan to coat the bottom, and cook for a few minutes until just set. Roll the omelette up and slide onto a plate. Cover with a second plate to keep it warm while you make the porridge.

⟫⟫ Put the oats and ginger in a saucepan with 1.2 litres/40fl oz/4¾ cups water. Bring to the boil over a high heat, then turn the heat down and simmer for 7–10 minutes, stirring regularly, until the oats are tender and most of the water has been absorbed. (You want the porridge to be marginally runnier than normal.) When almost cooked, stir in the miso and soy sauce.

⟫⟫ Slice the omelette into ribbons. Spoon the porridge into bowls, then top with the omelette, cashews and a sprinkling of nori flakes, if using.

Seed <u>AND</u> spice soda bread <u>WITH</u> fresh blueberry conserve

Soda bread is best eaten fresh on the day of baking, preferably when it's still warm, which is why I've divided the dough to make two loaves so one can be frozen until ready to eat. All you need to do is defrost the loaf and warm it in the oven before serving. However, if it suits you better, you can make one large loaf and bake it for 40–45 minutes. If you can't find buttermilk, replace it with plain yogurt with the addition of 1 teaspoon lemon juice.

⟩⟩⟩ Preheat the oven to 200°C/400°F/Gas 6. Dust a large baking sheet with flour.

⟩⟩⟩ Sift the flour into a large mixing bowl, adding any bran left in the sieve/fine-mesh strainer. Using a wooden spoon, stir in the bicarbonate of soda/baking soda, mixed spice/apple pie spice, seeds and salt and make a well in the middle.

⟩⟩⟩ Whisk together the buttermilk and egg, then stir them into the dry ingredients using a fork and then your hands to make a soft, slightly sticky dough. Add a little extra milk if the dough seems too dry. Tip the dough onto a lightly floured work surface, divide in half and gently knead each piece a couple of times to form them into round loaves. ⟩

MAKES ⟩⟩⟩ **2 SMALL LOAVES**
Preparation time ⟩ 15 minutes
Cooking time ⟩ 30 minutes

355g/12½oz/scant 3 cups wholemeal spelt or plain/all-purpose flour, plus extra for dusting
1 tsp bicarbonate of soda/baking soda
1 tbsp mixed spice/apple pie spice
5 tbsp mixed seeds, such as sunflower, pumpkin and flaxseed
1 tsp salt
185ml/6fl oz/¾ cup buttermilk
1 egg, lightly beaten
a little milk, if needed
unsalted butter, to serve

⟩⟩⟩ **Fresh blueberry conserve**
200g/7oz/1½ cups blueberries
1 tbsp caster/granulated sugar
1 tsp vanilla extract
1 tbsp lemon juice

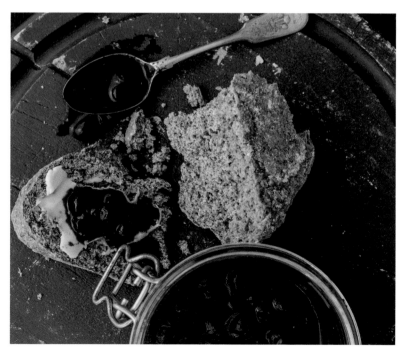

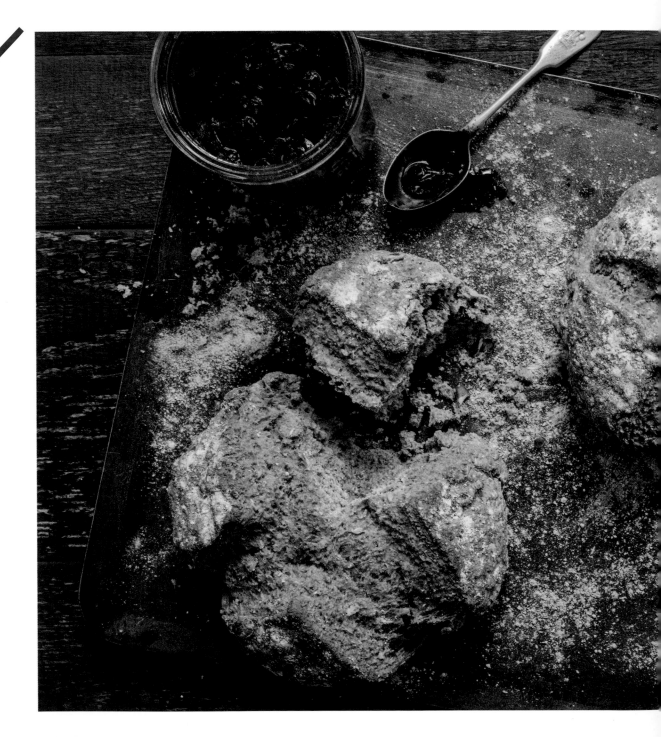

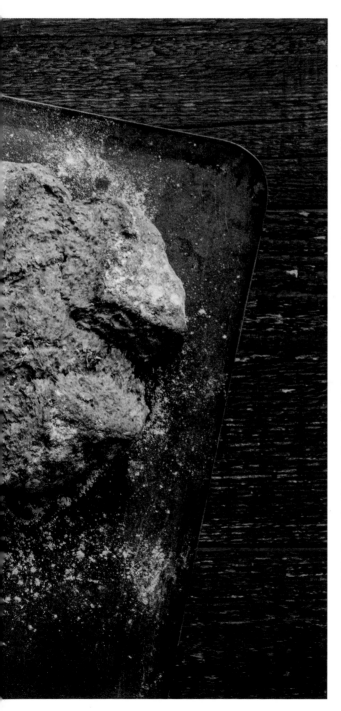

>>> Put the loaves onto the prepared baking sheet, sprinkle over a little extra flour and make a cross-shaped cut halfway down into the loaves. Bake for 30 minutes, or until risen and golden. Transfer to a wire rack to cool slightly.

>>> Meanwhile, make the conserve. Put the blueberries in a small heavy-based saucepan with the sugar, vanilla and lemon juice. Warm over a low heat, stirring, until the sugar dissolves and the blueberry juices start to run. Increase the heat and boil gently for 5 minutes, or until reduced to a jam consistency, crushing the blueberries slightly with the back of a fork.

>>> Serve the conserve spread on thick slices of fresh or toasted, buttered soda bread.

PART-TIME VARIATIONS

>>> Mixed fruit loaf

You could add fruit to the loaf instead of making a separate conserve: try 125g/4½oz/1 cup roughly chopped dried apricots, dates or raisins and stir in with the mixed spice/apple pie spice.

>>> Smoked mackerel pâté

For a savoury loaf, omit the spice and serve the soda bread topped with a meat, fish or vegetarian pâté. This simple smoked mackerel pâté is made by blending together 175g/6oz skinned smoked mackerel, 2 tbsp cream cheese and the juice of ½ lemon. Season with freshly ground black pepper, to taste. You could also make a smoked salmon pâté in the same way.

Butternut squash scones
WITH goats' cheese

MAKES ⟩⟩⟩ **8–10**

Preparation time ⟩ 15 minutes
Cooking time ⟩ 12 minutes

50g/1¾oz/3½ tbsp unsalted butter,
    plus extra for greasing
225g/8oz/1¾ cups self-raising/self-
    rising flour, plus extra for dusting
1 tsp baking powder
½ tsp salt
1 tbsp dried thyme
140g/5oz cooked, cooled and peeled
    butternut squash, coarsely grated
3 tbsp plain yogurt
1 tbsp milk, plus extra for brushing
mild, creamy goats' cheese, to serve

Scones may be synonymous with English tea but they're just as good for breakfast. The squash adds colour to these scones as well as keeping their texture moist and light. Steam rather than boil the squash before using and, once cooked, leave it to dry in its own heat before grating it into the dough mixture. Serve the scones with a generous filling of goats' cheese – I've opted for a relatively mild, creamy one.

⟩⟩⟩ Preheat the oven to 200°C/400°F/Gas 6 and grease and flour a baking sheet.

⟩⟩⟩ Mix together the flour, baking powder and salt in a large mixing bowl. Rub in the butter using your fingertips until the mixture resembles fine breadcrumbs, then stir in two-thirds of the thyme.

⟩⟩⟩ Mix together the squash, yogurt and milk, then gently stir the mixture into the dry ingredients using a wooden spoon, then gather the dough together into a ball.

⟩⟩⟩ Tip the dough out onto a lightly floured work surface, pat out to a 2cm/¾in thick round and score into 8 wedges. (Alternatively, use a 5cm/2in cutter to stamp out rounds. Lightly knead together any remnants of dough and stamp out more scones to make 10 in total.) Place on the prepared baking sheet.

⟩⟩⟩ Brush the top of the scones with a little extra milk and sprinkle with the remaining thyme. Bake for 10–12 minutes until risen and golden. Cool on a wire rack, then serve spread with a generous layer of goats' cheese.

PART-TIME VARIATION

⟩⟩⟩ **Sweet scones**

Stir 1 heaped tbsp caster/granulated sugar into the dry ingredients instead of the thyme and increase the quantity of milk to 100ml/3½fl oz/scant ½ cup in place of the butternut squash.

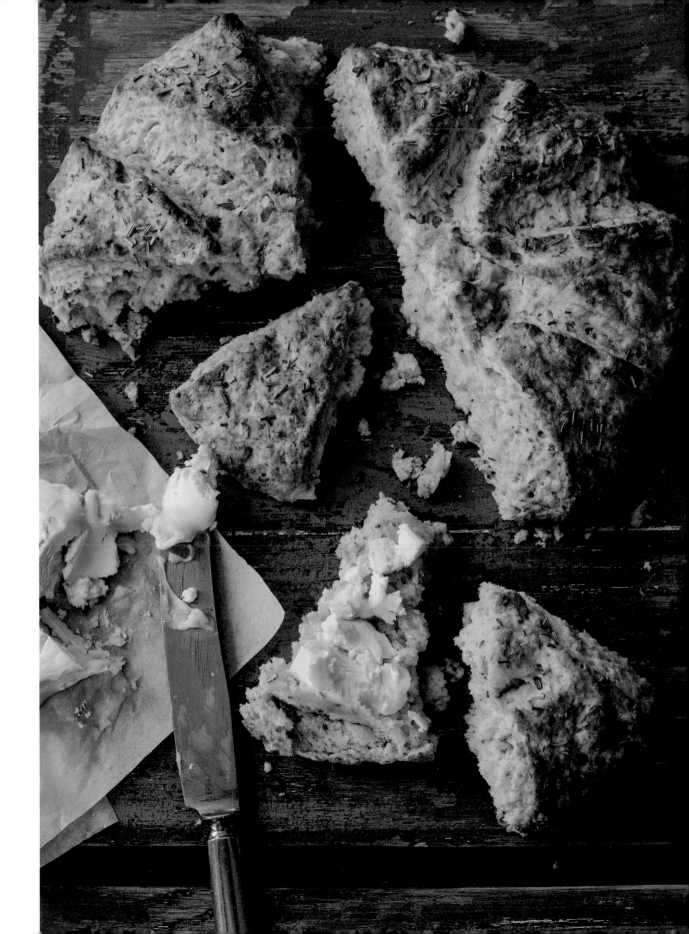

Sweetcorn muffins
WITH avocado salsa

MAKES ››› 6
Preparation time › 15 minutes
Cooking time › 30 minutes

70g/2½oz/4½ tbsp butter, melted, plus
    extra for greasing
125g/4½oz/1 cup self-raising/
    self-rising flour
50g/1¾oz/⅓ cup fine polenta/
    cornmeal
1 tsp English mustard powder
½ tsp salt
125g/4½oz/scant 1¼ cups canned
    drained sweetcorn
2 spring onions/scallions, finely
    chopped
1 large egg, lightly beaten
6 tbsp milk
1 red chilli, deseeded and finely
    chopped
1 recipe quantity Avocado Salsa
    (see page 66), to serve

Polenta, or cornmeal, adds a great colour and texture to these muffins, and thanks to the inclusion of self-raising/self-rising flour, they remain light. In keeping with the Mexican feel, the muffins come with a flavour-packed lime and avocado salsa.

››› Preheat the oven to 190°C/375°F/Gas 5 and lightly grease a 6-hole muffin pan or line with large muffin cases.

››› Sift together the flour, polenta/cornmeal, mustard powder and salt in a large mixing bowl, then mix until combined.

››› Put the sweetcorn and half the spring onions/scallions in a blender and blend to a coarse purée, then add the egg, milk and melted butter and blend again. Add this sweetcorn mixture to the dry ingredients with the remaining spring onions/scallions and the chilli and stir gently with a wooden spoon until just combined.

››› Spoon the sweetcorn batter into the muffin pan or cases and bake for 25–30 minutes until risen and golden.

››› Serve the muffins warm with the avocado salsa by the side.

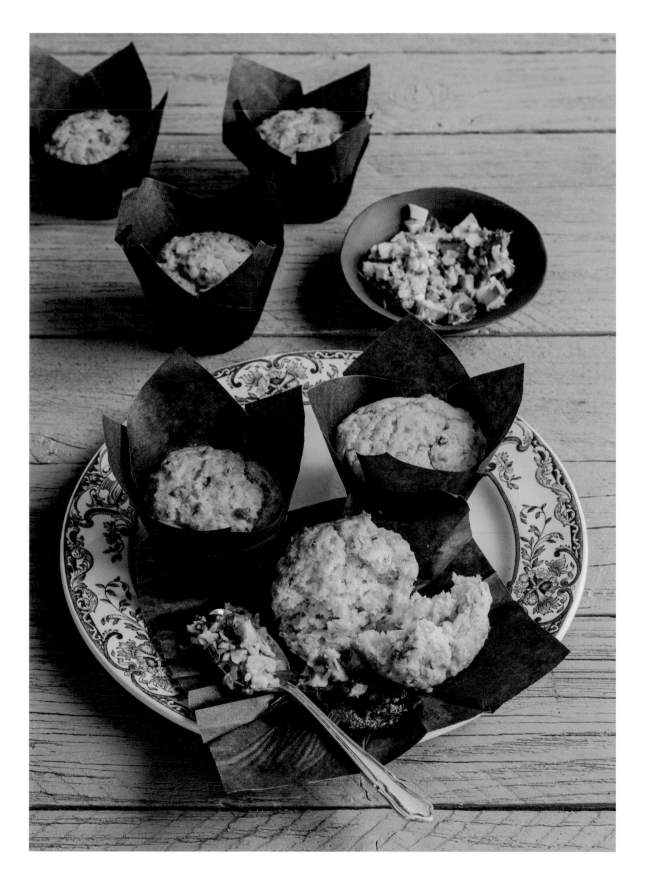

Pikelets <u>WITH</u> pear <u>AND</u> ginger compôte

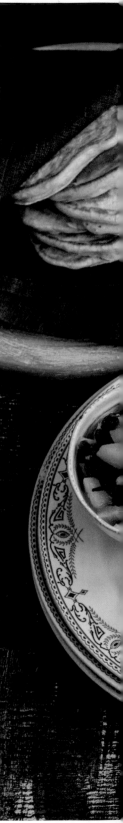

SERVES ⟩⟩⟩ 4

Preparation time ⟩ 15 minutes,
plus rising

Cooking time ⟩ 16 minutes

225g/8oz/1¾ cups plain/all-purpose
   flour, preferably spelt
1 tsp instant dried yeast
2 tsp caster/granulated sugar
1 large egg
270ml/9½fl oz/scant 1¼ cups milk
½ tsp salt
sunflower oil, for frying
Greek yogurt, to serve

⟩⟩⟩ **Pear and ginger compôte**

3 just-ripe pears, peeled, cored and
   cut into bite-size cubes
finely grated zest and juice of 1 orange
1cm/½in piece of fresh root ginger,
   peeled and finely chopped
6 cloves
40g/1½oz/⅓ cup sultanas/golden
   raisins
1–2 tbsp clear honey

A cross between the English crumpet and American pancake, the pikelet is said to have originated in Wales. You need to plan ahead when making pikelets as the yeast requires time to do its thing, so these are best served for brunch (or indeed for tea). They come with a warming pear compôte flavoured with ginger and cloves, but can also be served topped with a few rashers of crisp bacon and a drizzle of maple syrup, as opposite.

⟩⟩⟩ To make the pikelets, mix together the flour, yeast and sugar in a large mixing bowl until combined, then make a well in the middle.

⟩⟩⟩ Whisk the egg into the milk. Pour the mixture into the well and gradually draw in the flour, whisking to make a smooth batter. Cover the bowl with cling film/plastic wrap and leave for 2 hours in a warm place until bubbly and risen. Stir in the salt just before cooking, otherwise it will inhibit the yeast.

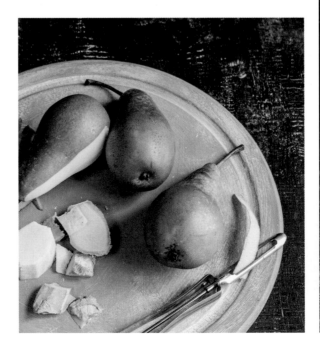

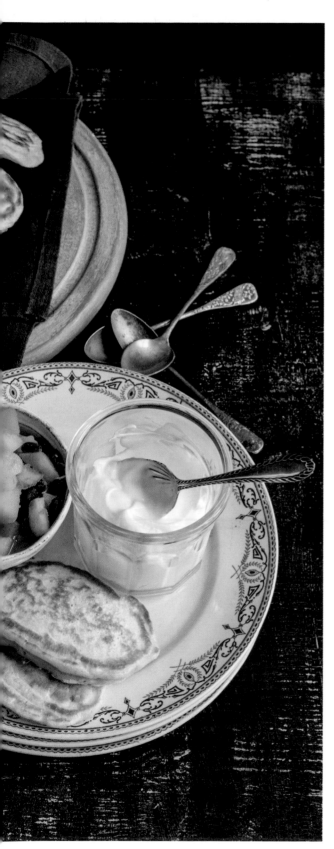

>>> Meanwhile, to make the compôte, put the pears, orange juice, ginger and cloves in a saucepan over a high heat and bring to the boil, then turn the heat down and stir in the orange zest and sultanas/golden raisins. Cover the pan and simmer for 5–8 minutes, or until the pears are just tender but not falling apart. Stir in enough honey to sweeten.

>>> Heat a little oil in a large non-stick frying pan over a medium heat and wipe it over the base using a crumpled up sheet of paper towel. Place a small ladleful (about 3 tablespoons) of the batter into the the pan, then repeat to cook 4 pikelets at a time. Cook for 2 minutes on each side, or until risen and golden. Keep warm wrapped in a cloth or in a low oven while you make the remaining pikelets.

>>> Serve the pikelets with the pear and ginger compôte and with yogurt on the side.

PART-TIME VARIATION

>>> Bacon and maple syrup pikelets

Pancakes and slices of crisp bacon are a classic combination, and pikelets work equally well. Preheat the grill/broiler to high and line the grill/broiler pan with foil. Grill/broil **8–12 rashers smoked streaky bacon** until crisp and golden. Drain on paper towels before serving on top of the pikelets with a **drizzle of maple syrup**.

Coconut AND cardamom pancakes WITH mango

SERVES ⟩⟩⟩ **4**

Preparation time ⟩ 15 minutes, plus resting

Cooking time ⟩ 10 minutes

175g/6oz/1⅓ cups plain/
   all-purpose flour
½ tsp salt
1 heaped tsp baking powder
2 tbsp caster/granulated sugar
1 tsp ground cinnamon, plus extra
   for sprinkling
2 eggs, lightly beaten
200ml/7fl oz/scant 1 cup dairy-free
   coconut milk (not canned)
seeds from 4 plump cardamom pods,
   ground
coconut or sunflower oil, for frying

⟩⟩⟩ **To serve**

1 large ripe mango, peeled, pitted
   and cubed
1 handful of pecans, toasted
   (see method on page 22)
maple syrup

Flavoured with coconut milk and spiced with cardamom and cinnamon, these American-style pancakes come with fresh mango and a sprinkling of pecan nuts. Canned coconut milk would be too rich for these pancakes, so use instead the ready-to-drink coconut milk found in most supermarkets alongside soya milk and the other dairy-free milk alternatives.

⟩⟩⟩ To make the batter, mix together the flour, salt, baking powder, sugar and cinnamon in a large mixing bowl until combined, then make a well in the middle.

⟩⟩⟩ Whisk the eggs into the coconut milk and stir in the ground cardamom seeds. Pour the mixture into the well and gradually draw in the flour mixture, whisking to make a smooth batter. Leave to rest for 15 minutes.

⟩⟩⟩ Melt enough coconut oil to lightly coat the base of a large non-stick frying pan over a medium heat. Place a small ladleful (about 3 tablespoons) of the batter into the pan, then repeat to cook 4 pancakes at a time. Cook for 2 minutes on each side, or until risen and golden. Keep warm wrapped in a cloth or in a low oven while you make the remaining pancakes.

⟩⟩⟩ Serve the pancakes with the mango, toasted pecans, a good drizzle of maple syrup and a dusting of extra cinnamon, if you like.

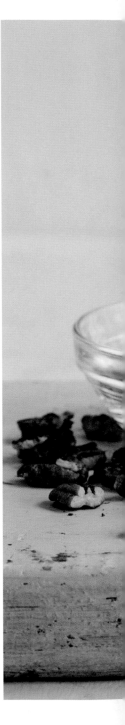

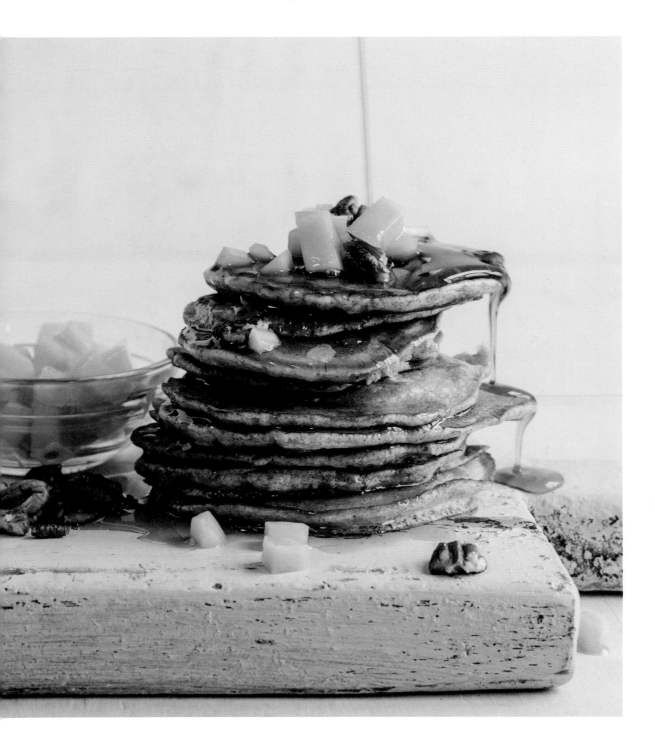

Olive AND tomato chickpea pancakes

SERVES ⟫⟫ **4**

Preparation time ⟩ 10 minutes, plus resting

Cooking time ⟩ 8 minutes

150g/5½oz/scant 1¼ cups gram/
   chickpea/besan flour

½ tsp salt

1 tsp harissa powder

1 large spring onion/scallion, finely
   chopped

1 handful of chopped coriander/
   cilantro leaves

sunflower oil, for frying

freshly ground black pepper

5 tbsp crème fraîche, to serve

⟫⟫ **Olive and tomato topping**

6 tomatoes, deseeded and diced

70g/2½oz/¾ cup pitted black olives,
   drained well and roughly chopped

4 tbsp chopped coriander/cilantro
   leaves

juice of ½ small lemon

These pancakes have more substance to them than, say, a French crêpe and also readily welcome added flavourings, such as herbs and spices. This is a great brunch to cater for all tastes as you can make the pancakes and then everyone can help themselves to the toppings, whether it be the olive and tomato or the marinated chicken, prawn/shrimp or lamb variations, opposite.

⟫⟫ Sift the chickpea flour into a large mixing bowl and stir in the salt and harissa, then make a well in the middle. Pour 270ml/9½fl oz/scant 1¼ cups water into the well and gradually draw in the flour mixture, whisking to make a smooth batter. Leave to rest for 30–60 minutes.

⟫⟫ Meanwhile, make the olive and tomato topping. Mix together the tomatoes, olives, coriander/cilantro and lemon juice, season, then leave to rest for 20 minutes.

⟫⟫ When the batter has rested, stir in the spring onion/scallion and a handful of coriander/cilantro, then season with pepper.

⟫⟫ Heat a large non-stick frying pan over a medium heat and add enough oil to lightly coat the base. Pour in one-quarter of the batter and tilt the pan so it lightly coats the base. Cook the pancake for 1 minute on each side, or until cooked and golden in places. Keep warm in a low oven while you cook the remaining pancakes, adding more oil each time. Serve the pancakes with a spoonful of crème fraîche and the tomato and olive mixture piled on top.

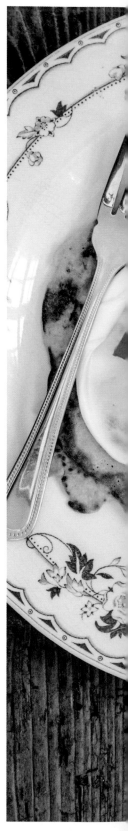

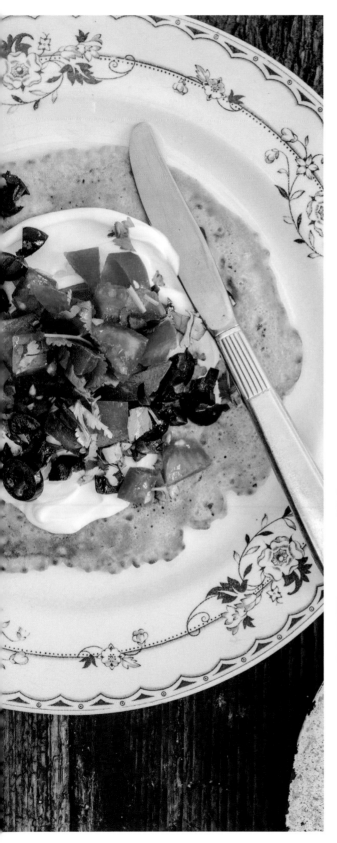

PART-TIME VARIATIONS

⟫⟫⟫ Chilli prawns/shrimp and chickpea pancakes

Go for 1 tsp nigella seeds and 1 finely chopped green chilli instead of the harissa in the batter. Serve with chilli-infused prawns/shrimp, cucumber raita and a spoonful of mango chutney.

⟫⟫⟫ Chicken or lamb chickpea pancakes

For a more substantial meal, top with slices of chargrilled tandoori chicken or yogurt and harissa-marinated strips of chargrilled lamb. Serve with a crisp green salad.

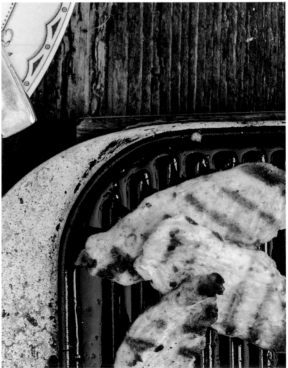

Hot mozzarella AND tapenade toasts

SERVES ⟩⟩⟩ 2

Preparation time ⟩ 15 minutes
Cooking time ⟩ 6 minutes

150ml/5fl oz/scant ⅔ cup milk
4 slices of good-quality white bread,
    crusts removed
100g/3½oz mozzarella cheese, patted
    dry and sliced
a few basil leaves, torn into pieces
2 tbsp olive oil

⟩⟩⟩ **Olive tapenade**

85g/3oz/scant 1 cup pitted green or
    black olives, drained
2 sun-dried tomatoes, roughly chopped
2 tbsp capers, rinsed and patted dry
1 garlic clove, crushed
2 tbsp extra virgin olive oil
1 large handful of flat-leaf parsley
    leaves
freshly ground black pepper

The secret to the success of this moreish breakfast toastie is to allow the mozzarella to melt sufficiently, but not so much that it escapes out of the sides. Home-made tapenade will happily keep in the refrigerator for up to 2 weeks and any leftovers would make a quick snack with warm pitta bread, or a speedy meal stirred into cooked pasta or spooned on top of a baked potato.

⟩⟩⟩ First make the tapenade. Put the olives in a food processor with the sun-dried tomatoes, capers, garlic, oil and parsley, then pulse briefly until finely chopped. Alternatively, coarsely chop all the ingredients by hand. Season with pepper and leave the tapenade to one side.

⟩⟩⟩ Pour the milk into a large shallow dish and dip one side of each slice of bread briefly in the mixture until wet but not soggy. Spread the non-milky side of two of the slices of bread with 1 tablespoon tapenade and scatter the mozzarella and basil on top. Top with the remaining bread, soaked-side out.

⟩⟩⟩ Heat the oil in a large non-stick frying pan over a medium heat and fry the sandwiches for 3 minutes on each side until golden and crisp, turning the heat down slightly if they brown too quickly. Remove from the pan and leave to stand for 1 minute to cool slightly. Cut each sandwich into fingers and serve straightaway. (Place any remaining tapenade in an airtight jar and pour a little extra oil over to cover. Secure with a lid and store in the refrigerator for up to 2 weeks.)

PART-TIME VARIATION
⟩⟩⟩ Ham and mozzarella toasts

Try adding a **slice of good-quality ham** to each 'sandwich' instead of the tapenade in step 2 if you are looking to serve the toasts to non-veggies.

Fried bread <u>WITH</u> kale, mushroom <u>AND</u> bean pan-fry

This is more delicious than the title may at first suggest – after all, what's not to like about fried bread? A runny yolk on your fried egg is a must, so when it's cut into it oozes over the kale, mushrooms and beans. For a vegan version of this weekend brunch, top with a generous spoonful of humous instead of the egg, or for a seafood alternative see the variation, below.

>>> Steam the kale for 2 minutes, or until just tender.

>>> Meanwhile, heat 2 tablespoons of the oil in a large non-stick frying pan over a medium heat and fry the bread for 3 minutes on each side, or until golden and crisp. Remove the fried bread from the pan, drain on paper towels and cover with foil to keep warm.

>>> Add the remaining oil to the frying pan with the mushrooms and beans and sauté for 4 minutes until tender, then stir in the steamed kale and lemon juice and season to taste with salt and pepper.

>>> While the vegetables and beans are cooking, heat enough oil to cover the base of a second frying pan over a medium heat and when hot, crack in the eggs, one by one. Fry the eggs, occasionally spooning the hot oil over the yolks so that they cook evenly. Cook for a few minutes until the white of each egg is cooked but the yolks remain runny. To serve, place a slice of fried bread on each plate. Top with the bean mixture, a fried egg and a spoonful of sweet chilli sauce.

PART-TIME VARIATION

>>> King prawn/jumbo shrimp pan-fry

Steam the kale as described above. Add **225g/8oz raw peeled king prawns/ jumbo shrimp** to the frying pan with the mushrooms and beans and continue as instructed above. Serve on the fried bread and top with the sweet chilli sauce, omitting the fried eggs.

SERVES >>> **4**

Preparation time ⟩ 5 minutes
Cooking time ⟩ 15 minutes

3 large handfuls of curly kale, tough
    stalks removed and leaves torn
    into large bite-size pieces
3 tbsp cold-pressed rapeseed/canola
    oil, plus extra for frying
4 large thick slices of sourdough or
    crusty bread
200g/7oz chestnut/cremini mushrooms,
    sliced
400g/14oz can cannellini beans, drained
    and rinsed
juice of ½ lemon
4 large eggs
sea salt and freshly ground black
    pepper
4 heaped tsp sweet chilli sauce, to
    serve

Parmesan French toast
<u>WITH</u> balsamic tomatoes

SERVES ››› 4

Preparation time › 10 minutes
Cooking time › 13 minutes

5 eggs, lightly beaten
5 tbsp milk
5 tbsp finely grated Parmesan cheese
4 large thick slices of country-style
    bread
sea salt and freshly ground black
    pepper
4 handfuls of rocket/arugula leaves and
    4 heaped tbsp curd cheese or
    cream cheese, to serve

››› Balsamic tomatoes

2 tsp olive oil
60g/2¼oz/4 tbsp butter
4 handfuls of cherry tomatoes
1 tbsp balsamic vinegar

A family favourite – you can't go far wrong with French toast. This savoury version is made more substantial with the topping of fried balsamic tomatoes, rocket/arugula and a spoonful of curd cheese, while you may like to add slices of crisp Parma ham for non-vegetarians. For a sweet alternative, flavour the egg mixture with a teaspoonful each of vanilla extract, icing/confectioners' sugar and ground cinnamon and top with fresh fruit and a little maple syrup.

››› Whisk the eggs, milk and Parmesan together in a large shallow dish and season with salt and pepper. Dunk both sides of each slice of bread in the egg mixture and leave to soak until needed.

››› To prepare the tomatoes, heat the oil and one-third of the butter in a large non-stick frying pan over a medium heat. Add the tomatoes, take care as they can splutter, and cook for 2–3 minutes until softened slightly, turning once. Pour in the balsamic vinegar and turn the tomatoes in the mixture for 1–2 minutes until slightly caramelized. Season with salt and pepper, then remove the tomatoes and any juices from the pan and keep warm in a low oven, covered to prevent them drying out.

››› Wipe the pan clean with paper towels, then add the remaining butter. When melted, add the egg-soaked bread, and cook for about 2 minutes on each side until golden and slightly crisp. (You may need to cook the bread in two batches.)

››› Place the Parmesan toasts on serving plates and top with the rocket/arugula, balsamic tomatoes and curd cheese. Finish with a grinding of black pepper and serve straightaway.

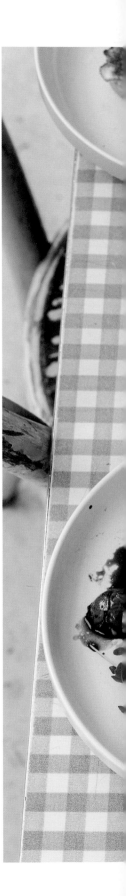

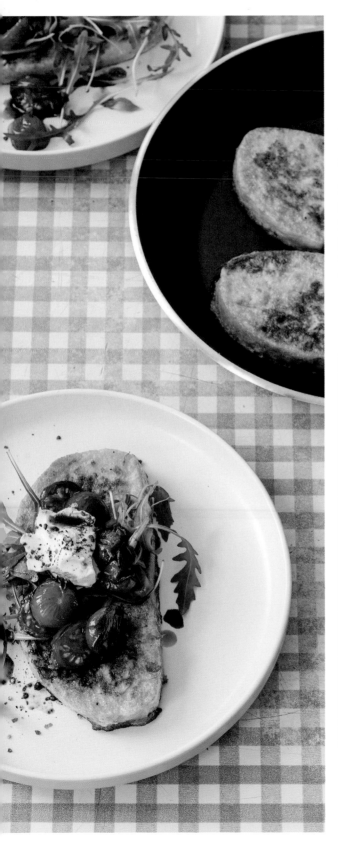

PART-TIME VARIATION
»»» French toast with Parma ham

Place **4–8 slices of Parma ham**, depending on their size, in the dry non-stick frying pan and cook over a medium heat for 3–4 minutes, turning once, until crisp. Remove from the pan and drain on paper towels while you cook the French toast. Serve on top of the Parmesan toast instead of, or as well as, the curd cheese.

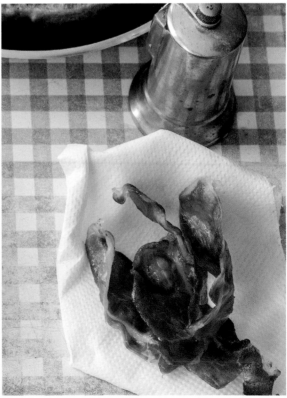

SPREADS, BUTTERS & KETCHUPS

Within each chapter of this book, you'll find a featured selection of mini recipes that at first glance may appear quite random, but they have all been chosen to enhance, embellish or complement the main recipes in one way or another.

The following recipes for sweet and savoury condiments and accompaniments are no exception and make a welcome alternative to shop-bought versions. For instance, you won't find any unwelcome additives, sugar or palm oil in the Almond and Cashew Butter. This nutritious nut spread is not only delicious on toast but can be used as a base for smoothies and sweet and savoury sauces. The Red Pepper Ketchup is equally versatile and makes a refreshing change to the more usual tomato-based one. Serve as an accompaniment to a fry-up, as a dip with flatbreads or as a sauce with pasta.

For a touch of sweetness, try the fruity Apricot and Vanilla Spread and Spiced Date and Apple Jam. Stir a good spoonful into smoothies or plain yogurt, or use as a topping for toast, pancakes, waffles or sweet scones.

⟫⟫ Apricot and vanilla spread

Put 200g/7oz/1½ cups roughly chopped unsulphured dried apricots in a saucepan with 300ml/10½fl oz/1¼ cups water. Bring to the boil over a high heat, then turn the heat down to low and simmer for 20 minutes, covered, until very soft and most of the water has been absorbed. Stir in 1 tsp vanilla extract and blend using a stick/immersion blender until smooth, adding a splash of water if the spread is too thick. Store in an airtight container in the refrigerator for up to 2 weeks.

⟫⟫ Spiced date and apple jam

Put 200g/7oz/1½ cups roughly chopped dried dates, 1 peeled, grated and cored apple, 1 tsp ground cinnamon and 1 tsp ground allspice in a saucepan with 300ml/10½fl oz/1¼ cups water. Bring to the boil over a high heat, then turn the heat down to low and simmer for 20 minutes, covered, until very soft and most of the water has been absorbed. Blend using a stick/immersion blender until smooth, adding a splash of water if the jam is too thick. Store in an airtight container in the refrigerator for up to 2 weeks.

››› Almond and cashew butter

Preheat the oven to 180°C/350°F/Gas 4. Put **100g/3½oz/¾ cup blanched almonds** and **50g/1¾oz/scant ½ cup cashews** in a large roasting pan and cook for 10–12 minutes, turning once, until the nuts start to colour and smell toasted. Transfer to a food processor and process to a fairly smooth, thick, creamy paste. Be patient as it can take a little time and you'll need to stir the mixture occasionally. Add **a good pinch of sea salt** and **1 tbsp cold-pressed rapeseed or melted coconut oil** (or other mild-tasting oil) and blend briefly until combined. Store in an airtight container in the refrigerator for up to 2 weeks.

››› Red pepper ketchup

A cross between a ketchup and a dip, this recipe is based on *ajvar* (pronounced 'eye-var'), which surprisingly originates from Eastern Europe, despite its Middle Eastern nuance. First, preheat the grill/broiler to high and line a grill/broiler pan with foil. Brush **1 aubergine/eggplant** and **2 large red peppers** with olive oil and grill/broil for 15 minutes, turning occasionally, until blackened all over. Turn the grill/broiler to the oven setting, if you have a combined model, and heat to 200°C/400°F/Gas 6. Put the aubergine/eggplant and pepper in a roasting pan and roast for 30 minutes until very tender. Put the peppers in a bowl and cover with cling film/plastic wrap. Scoop the aubergine/eggplant flesh, discarding any seeds, into a food processor. Peel and discard the seeds from the peppers, then put the flesh and juices in the food processor. Add **1 crushed garlic clove, 1 tsp mild smoked paprika** and **2 tbsp white wine vinegar** and blend until smooth. Season with sea salt and store in an airtight container in the refrigerator for up to a week.

Poached eggs WITH rainbow chard AND lemon hollandaise

SERVES ⟩⟩⟩ 4
Preparation time ⟩ 15 minutes
Cooking time ⟩ 10 minutes

100g/3½oz rainbow chard, stems
    and leaves separated and sliced
1 tsp white wine vinegar
4 large eggs
sea salt and freshly ground black
    pepper
4 toasted English muffins, split open,
    to serve

⟩⟩⟩ **Lemon hollandaise**
2 egg yolks
1½ tbsp lemon juice
100g/3½oz/7 tbsp butter, melted
1 tsp finely grated lemon zest

A twist on the classic eggs Florentine, this uses stunning rainbow chard with its golden and magenta stems and vibrant green and burgandy leaves. The chard is topped with a poached egg and a simple lemony hollandaise sauce. Curly kale, cavolo nero or the more usual spinach are all good substitutes for the chard.

⟩⟩⟩ To make the hollandaise, heat 5cm/2in water in a saucepan to simmering point. Place a heatproof bowl over the pan, making sure the bottom doesn't touch the water. Turn the heat to low and whisk together the egg yolks, lemon juice and 1 tablespoon warm water in the bowl until combined. Gradually, add the melted butter, whisking continuously, to make a smooth, creamy sauce and adding a little more warm water, if needed. Season with salt and pepper to taste, and stir in the lemon zest. Remove from the heat and cover to keep warm.

⟩⟩⟩ Meanwhile, add the chard stalks to a steamer and steam for 1 minute, then add the leaves and cook for another 2 minutes, or until tender. Drain well.

⟩⟩⟩ To poach the eggs, bring a large sauté pan of water to the boil over a high heat and add the vinegar, then turn the heat down to a gentle simmer. Crack an egg into a ramekin. Swirl the water, then gently slip the egg into the water and begin to time 3 minutes. Add the remaining eggs to the water in the same way and poach the eggs for 3 minutes, or until the whites are just set but the yolks remain runny. Lift the eggs out of the water using a slotted spoon in the order you put them in, then drain well.

⟩⟩⟩ Place the chard on top of the toasted muffins, followed by the poached eggs and the lemon hollandaise.

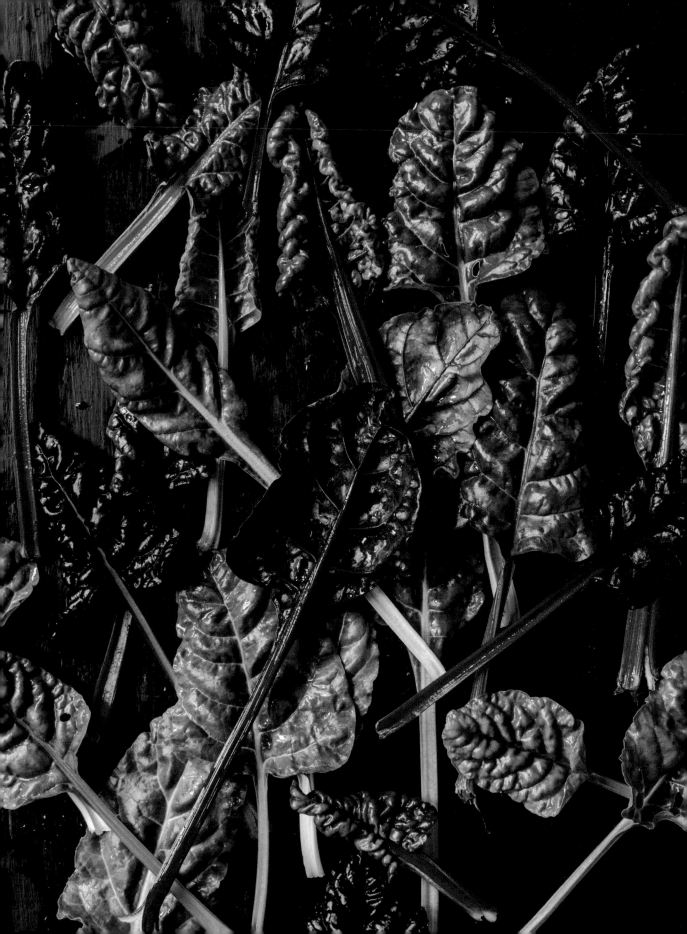

Egg pots <u>WITH</u> asparagus dippers

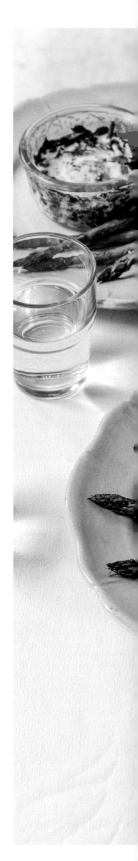

SERVES ⟩⟩⟩ 4

Preparation time ⟩ 10 minutes

Cooking time ⟩ 17 minutes

200g/7oz baby leaf spinach, tough
    stalks removed

butter, for greasing

3 tbsp finely grated Parmesan cheese

4 large eggs

4 tbsp double/heavy cream

250g/9oz asparagus spears, ends
    trimmed

olive oil, for brushing

sea salt and freshly ground black
    pepper

toast fingers, to serve

A simple weekend breakfast for friends or family, this recipe makes the most of the heat of the oven by roasting the asparagus at the same time as baking the eggs. It is also an easy dish to adapt to all tastes as in the Crab Egg Pots, opposite, or you could use chopped ham or chorizo and tomato. The asparagus is perfect for dunking into the runny egg yolks.

⟩⟩⟩ Preheat the oven to 190°C/375°F/Gas 5. Steam the spinach for 2 minutes until wilted, then drain well and squeeze to remove any excess water. Roughly chop the spinach and leave to one side.

⟩⟩⟩ Meanwhile, liberally grease 4 large ramekins with butter and sprinkle the Parmesan over the base and up the sides of each one. Spoon the spinach into the ramekins and crack in an egg. Pour a tablespoonful of cream on top and season with salt and pepper. Bake for 12–15 minutes until the whites are set but the yolks remain runny.

⟩⟩⟩ Meanwhile, brush the asparagus with a little oil, put them in a roasting pan and roast for 10 minutes, turning once, until just tender. Serve the egg pots with the asparagus and fingers of toast by the side.

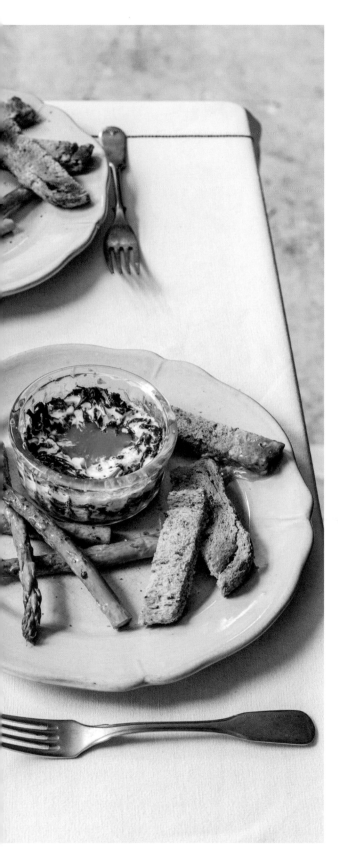

PART-TIME VARIATION
»»» Crab egg pots

Fresh crabmeat makes an indulgent alternative to the spinach and Parmesan. Divide **100g/3½oz fresh white and brown crabmeat** among the ramekins. Top with the egg and cream, then bake as instructed. Alternatively, try a similar quantity of **smoked salmon** – the off-cuts that you can buy are ideal.

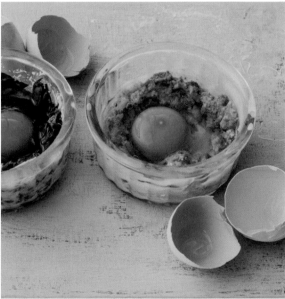

Breakfast tortillas

SERVES ⟩⟩⟩ **4**

Preparation time ⟩ 10 minutes
Cooking time ⟩ 30 minutes

1 tbsp butter, plus extra for greasing
1 onion, finely chopped
2 cooked potatoes (about 250g/9oz
    total weight), such as Maris Piper,
    peeled and cut into large cubes
4 large eggs, lightly beaten
2 tbsp double/heavy cream or milk
3 tbsp snipped chives
4 cherry tomatoes, halved
sea salt and freshly ground black
    pepper

Quick to prepare, these individual tortillas are baked in a muffin pan. If liked, you could easily make one half of them vegetarian and the other half with bacon – see the variation, below, reducing the quantity of bacon to three rashers. Why not make the most of the heat of the oven by roasting extra cherry tomatoes at the same time as cooking the tortillas to serve as an accompaniment?

⟩⟩⟩ Preheat the oven to 180°C/350°C/Gas 4. Liberally grease 8 holes in a muffin pan with butter.

⟩⟩⟩ Melt the remaining butter in a large non-stick frying pan over a medium heat and cook the onion for 8 minutes, stirring regularly, until softened. Stir in the cooked potatoes and cook for another 2 minutes until warmed though.

⟩⟩⟩ Meanwhile, whisk together the eggs, cream and chives in a large mixing bowl and season with salt and pepper. Stir in the onion mixture until combined, then ladle into the prepared muffin pan. Place a half of tomato on top of each tortilla and bake for 15–18 minutes until risen and just set.

PART-TIME VARIATION
⟩⟩⟩ Bacon breakfast tortillas

Dice 6 rashers smoked streaky bacon and fry in 1 tbsp olive oil for 5 minutes, or until crisp. Remove from the pan and drain on paper towels. Pour off all but 1 tbsp of the fat in the pan before you cook the onion. Continue as described above, omitting the chives.

Smoked paprika, tomato AND herb scramble

For the best-tasting scramble, try to use organic, free-range eggs. However, the way the eggs are cooked is also crucial as you need to keep an eye on time and the level of heat to avoid a dry, over-cooked scramble. It's best to keep the heat low and stir gently but often for soft, creamy curds.

>>> Preheat the oven to 130°C/250°F/Gas 1. Wrap the tortillas in foil and place in the oven to warm for 5 minutes.

>>> Meanwhile, melt the butter in a saucepan over a medium heat. Add the tomatoes and spring onions/scallions and cook for 2 minutes, stirring regularly. Turn the heat down to low and stir in half the coriander/cilantro.

>>> Break the eggs into a bowl, add the milk and season with smoked paprika and salt. Whisk until combined and pour into the pan. Cook for 3–5 minutes, turning the eggs gently but continuously with a spatula until cooked into large 'flakes'. Serve on top of the warm tortillas, sprinkled with the remaining coriander/cilantro.

PART-TIME VARIATION
>>> Smoked salmon scramble

Smoked salmon and scrambled eggs is a classic combination. Instead of serving them separately, stir 125g/4½oz smoked salmon or trout pieces into the eggs towards the end of their cooking time and allow to warm through and become opaque. Omit the tomatoes, spring onions/scallions, coriander/cilantro and paprika and serve on top of toasted brioche sprinkled with 2 tbsp snipped chives, a grinding of black pepper and a squeeze of lemon juice instead.

SERVES >>> 4

Preparation time > 10 minutes
Cooking time > 5 minutes

4 small soft corn or wheat tortillas
70g/2½oz/4½ tbsp butter
5 vine-ripened tomatoes, deseeded
    and diced
4 spring onions/scallions, finely
    chopped
4 tbsp roughly chopped coriander/
    cilantro leaves
8 large eggs, lightly beaten
6 tbsp milk
½ tsp hot smoked paprika
sea salt

Home-style baked beans
WITH roasted portabellini

SERVES ⟩⟩⟩ **4**
Preparation time ⟩ 5 minutes
Cooking time ⟩ 12 minutes

3 tbsp olive oil
2 x 400g/14oz cans haricot beans,
    drained
4 good-size vine tomatoes, deseeded
    and diced
6 tbsp tomato purée/paste
2 tbsp dark soy sauce
sea salt and freshly ground black
    pepper

⟩⟩⟩ **To serve**
300g/10½oz portabellini mushrooms
2 tbsp chopped flat-leaf parsley leaves
thick slices of buttered toast

These beans take just minutes to rustle up and are so much better than the canned alternative. Top them with roasted portabellini mushrooms and a sprinkling of parsley – a fried egg wouldn't go amiss either, or some diced chorizo.

⟩⟩⟩ Preheat the oven to 200°C/400°F/Gas 6. Put one-third of the oil, the beans, tomatoes, tomato purée/paste, soy sauce and 4 tablespoons water in a saucepan and warm over a medium heat. When the mixture almost reaches boilng point, turn the heat down slightly and simmer for 10 minutes, covered, until the beans are tender and the sauce has thickened. Season with salt and pepper to taste – but go easy on the salt bearing in mind that the soy sauce is salty.

⟩⟩⟩ Meanwhile, brush the mushrooms with the remaining oil. Season with salt and pepper, put in a roasting pan and put in the oven for 8 minutes until tender. Serve the mushrooms, sprinkled with parsley, on top of the beans, with buttered toast by the side.

PART-TIME VARIATION
⟩⟩⟩ Chorizo baked beans

Add 140g/5oz diced chorizo or 200g/7oz smoked hot cooking chorizo with the beans, following the cooking instructions, above. Serve sprinkled with chopped coriander/cilantro on slices of buttered toast, instead of the roasted mushrooms and parsley.

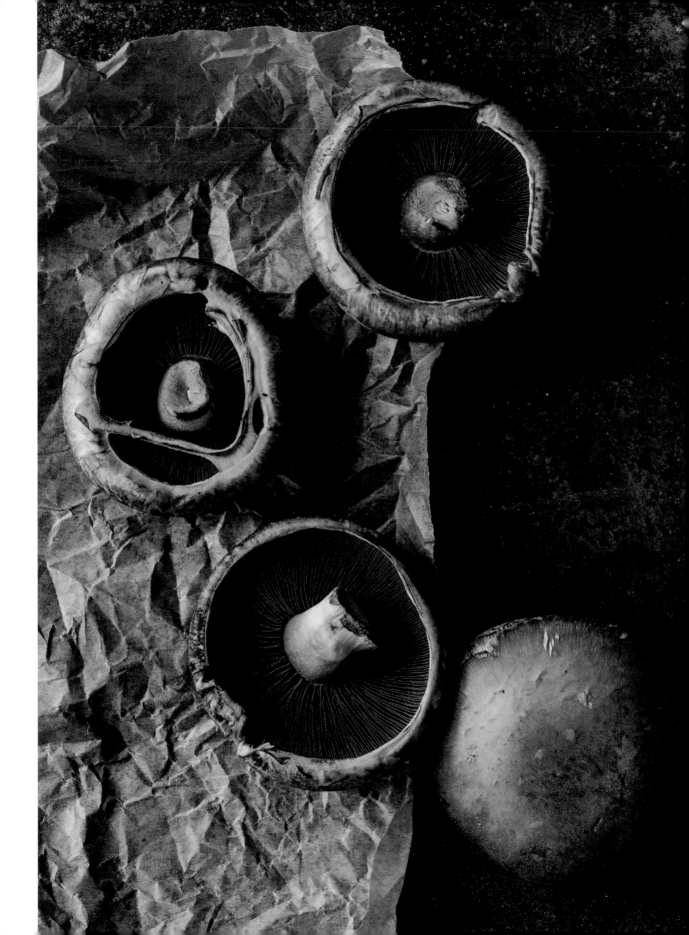

Halloumi hash

SERVES ⟩⟩⟩ **4**

Preparation time ⟩ 10 minutes

Cooking time ⟩ 10 minutes

2 tbsp olive oil

250g/9oz halloumi cheese, rinsed,
  patted dry and cut into
  1cm/½in cubes

4 good-size roast potatoes or
  8 cooked new potatoes, cubed

250g/9oz cooked Brussels sprouts,
  halved

250g/9oz cooked green hispi or Savoy
  cabbage, shredded

4 handfuls of cherry tomatoes

1 tsp cumin seeds

½ tsp dried chilli/hot pepper flakes

1cm/½in piece of fresh root ginger,
  peeled and finely chopped

1 large garlic clove, finely chopped

If you have any leftover roasties or cooked vegetables, then this dish is the perfect way to use them up. Don't feel restricted by my choice of vegetables. Utilize any leftovers you have to hand within reason. The halloumi adds an interesting twist to this old favourite but, if sticking to the leftover theme, it's also a good way of using up roast meat. If you don't have any leftovers, this brunch is worthy of cooking the vegetables from scratch.

⟩⟩⟩ Heat half the oil in a large non-stick sauté pan over a medium heat and sauté the halloumi for 2–3 minutes, turning occasionally, until starting to colour. Remove from the pan with a slotted spoon and leave to one side.

⟩⟩⟩ Add the remaining oil to the pan, turn the heat up slightly and add the cooked potatoes, sprouts and cabbage. Stir-fry for 3 minutes until starting to colour and crisp.

⟩⟩⟩ Turn the heat to medium, add the tomatoes, cumin, chilli/hot pepper flakes, ginger and garlic and stir-fry for 2 minutes until the tomatoes have softened slightly. Return the halloumi to the pan to heat through, then serve.

PART-TIME VARIATIONS

⟩⟩⟩ Roast meat hash

Make use of leftover roast meat – including chicken, pork, lamb or beef – instead of the halloumi. Cut **200g/7oz roast meat** into bite-size pieces and add with the tomatoes in the final step to heat through.

⟩⟩⟩ Salmon hash

Alternatively, swap the halloumi for fresh salmon. Preheat the grill/broiler to high and line the grill/broiler pan with foil. Season **2 large skinless salmon fillets** with salt and pepper. Cut each fillet crossways into 4 thick slices and place on the foil. Grill/broil for 2 minutes, turning once, or until just cooked. Place on top of the cooked vegetables before serving.

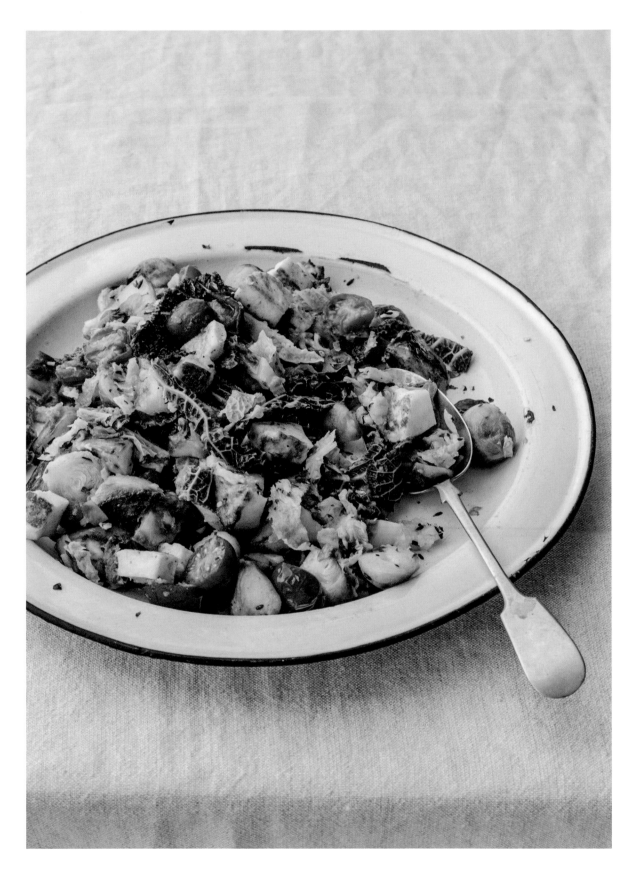

Kosheri

SERVES ⟫⟫ **4**

Preparation time ⟩ 15 minutes
Cooking time ⟩ 25 minutes

200g/7oz/heaped 1 cup brown
   basmati rice, rinsed
1 tsp turmeric
6 cloves
4 cardamom pods, split
2 tsp vegetable bouillon powder
1 heaped tbsp medium curry powder
juice of 1 small lemon
60g/2¼oz/⅓ cup split red lentils, rinsed
sea salt and freshly ground black
   pepper

⟫⟫ **To serve**

40g/1½oz/2½ tbsp butter
2 onions, finely sliced
2.5cm/1in piece of fresh root ginger,
   peeled and cut into thin strips
4 tbsp thick plain yogurt
4 hard-boiled eggs, quartered
1 handful of chopped coriander/
   cilantro leaves

Red lentils are stirred into spiced basmati rice to make this filling, traditional Indian breakfast, which has many similarities to the classic kedgeree. Top the kosheri with quartered hard-boiled eggs for a more substantial brunch.

⟫⟫ Put the rice in a saucepan and pour in enough water to cover by 1.5cm/⅝in. Stir in the turmeric, cloves and cardamom and bring to the boil over a high heat, then stir in the vegetable bouillon. Turn the heat down to very low, cover and simmer for 25 minutes, or until the rice is cooked and the water has been absorbed. Stir in the curry powder and lemon juice, turn off the heat, and leave to sit for about 5 minutes, covered.

⟫⟫ Meanwhile, put the lentils in a separate pan, cover generously with water and bring to the boil over a high heat. Turn the heat down to low, part-cover, and simmer for 15 minutes, or until tender, scooping off any foam that rises to the surface. Drain the lentils, then stir them into the spiced rice mixture and season with salt and pepper to taste.

⟫⟫ While the rice and lentils are cooking, melt the butter in a large non-stick frying pan over a medium heat and fry the onions for 8 minutes, then add the ginger and cook for another 2 minutes until softened and starting to turn golden. Serve the onions and ginger on top of the rice mixture with the yogurt and quartered hard-boiled eggs, then sprinkle with coriander/cilantro.

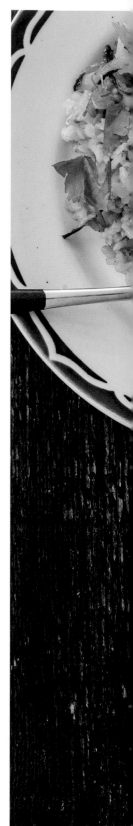

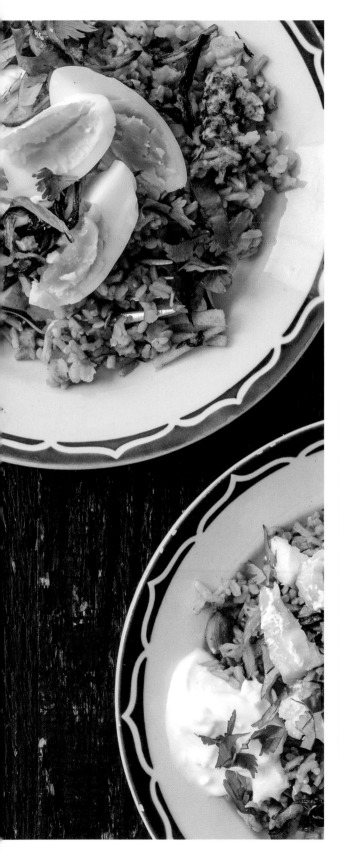

PART-TIME VARIATION
››› Smoked haddock kedgeree

Put **450g/1lb undyed smoked haddock** in a large sauté pan and cover with water. Bring almost to the boil, then turn the heat down to low and simmer gently for 5 minutes, or until the haddock is just cooked and opaque. Using a spatula, remove the fish from the pan to a plate and peel away the skin and pick out any bones. Flake the fish into large pieces and stir it into the rice just before serving to warm through. Serve the fish in place of the lentils and hard-boiled eggs.

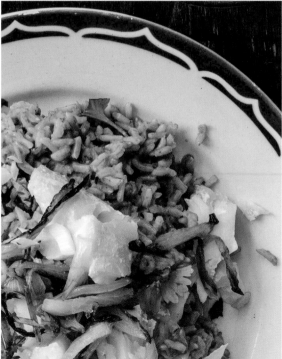

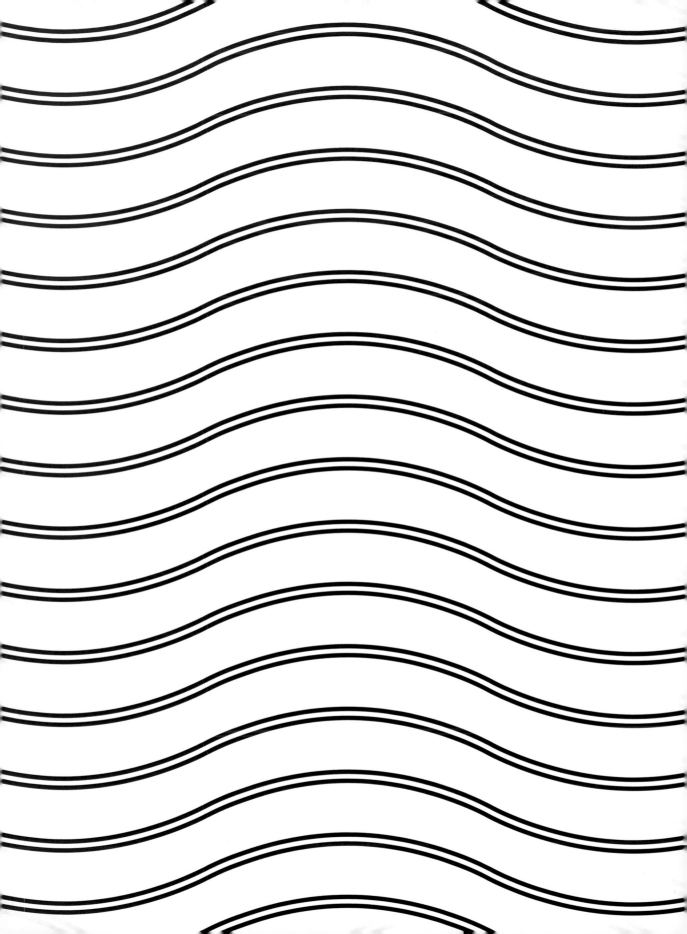

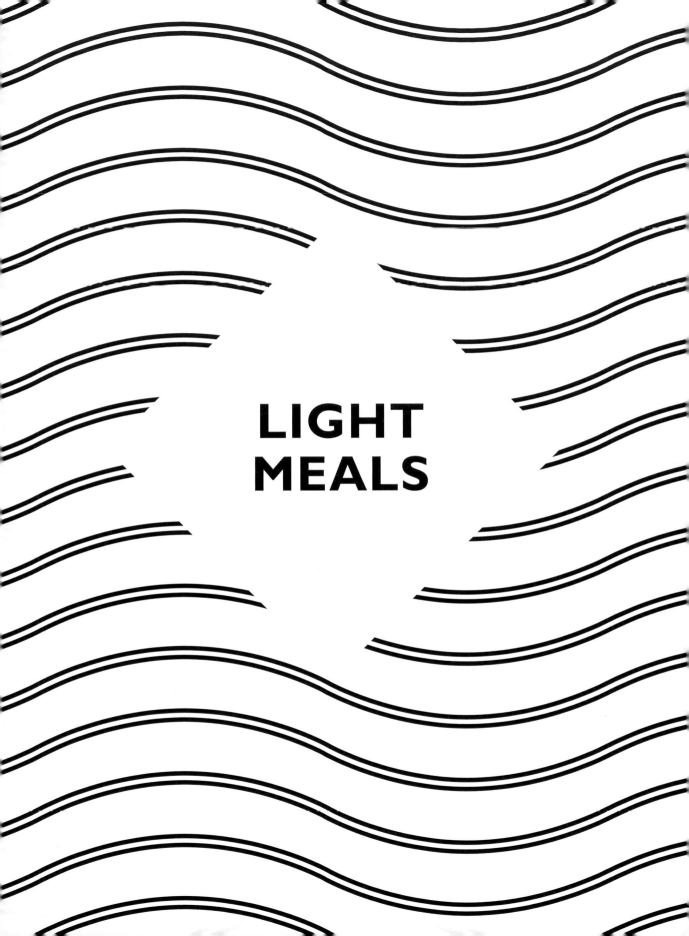

LIGHT MEALS

Avocado gazpacho

SERVES ››› 4

Preparation time ⟩ 15 minutes

3 spring onions/scallions, sliced

1 large ripe avocado, pitted and flesh
   scooped out

1 small cucumber, deseeded and
   chopped

115g/4oz/¾ cup frozen peas

400ml/14fl oz/1¾ cups cold vegetable
   stock, plus extra if needed

juice of 1 lime

2 tsp yuzu juice or extra lime
   or lemon juice

1 green chilli, deseeded and
   thinly sliced

1 large handful of coriander/cilantro
   leaves, plus extra to serve

a splash of hot pepper sauce

››› To serve

8 ice cubes

2 vine-ripened tomatoes, deseeded
   and diced

extra virgin olive oil

corn chips

If you're looking for a healthy dish to serve to friends for a snack or light lunch, then this is perfect and you could even make some bresaola crisps (see below) for non-vegetarian guests. Though not in keeping with the 'Mexican' feel of this recipe, the yuzu juice lifts the flavour of the thick and creamy soup-cum-smoothie – does that make it a smoopie? You can now buy the juice in Asian grocers and the speciality section of some large supermarkets.

››› Reserve a little of the green part of the spring onions/scallions to serve, then put the remainder in a blender with the avocado, cucumber, peas, stock, lime juice, yuzu, chilli and coriander/cilantro and blend until smooth, thick and creamy. The gazpacho should be the consistency of a runny smoothie, so add extra stock, if needed. Stir in a splash of hot pepper sauce, then put it in the refrigerator for 30 minutes to chill.

››› To serve, pour into glasses or bowls, add the ice cubes and top with the tomatoes, extra chopped coriander/cilantro leaves, reserved spring onions/scallions and a drizzle of olive oil. Serve with the corn chips by the side.

PART-TIME VARIATION
››› Avocado gazpacho with bresaola crisps

Top the avocado gazpacho with crisp shards of bresaola or Parma ham. To cook, put **4–8 thin slices bresaola** or **Parma ham** in a dry, non-stick frying pan and cook for a few minutes, turning once, until crisp. Leave to cool, then break into pieces before sprinkling on top of the gazpacho in place of the tomato.

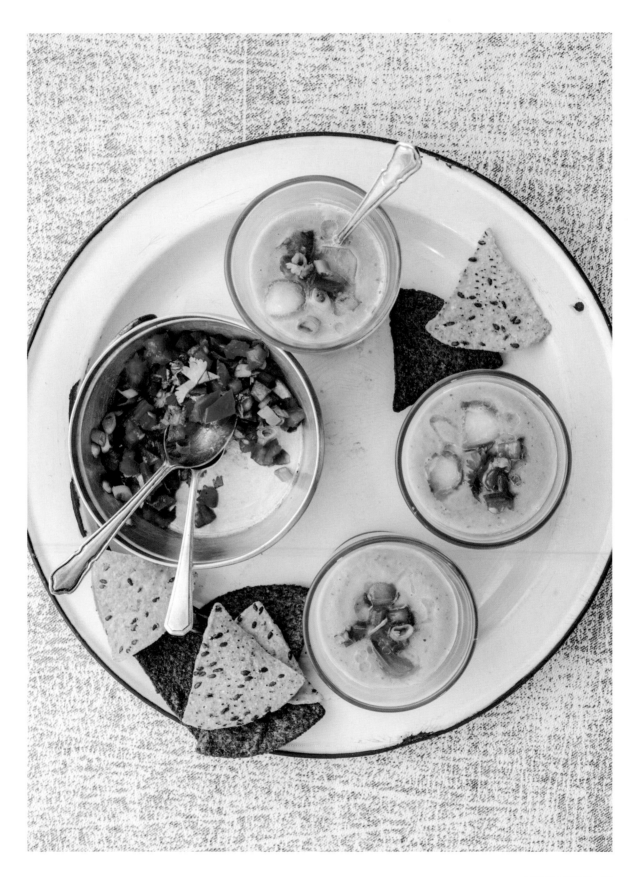

Beetroot soup <u>WITH</u> spiced orange yogurt

SERVES ⟫⟫ **4–6**

Preparation time ⟩ 15 minutes
Cooking time ⟩ 40 minutes

1 tbsp olive oil
1 large onion, chopped
2 carrots, sliced
1 celery stalk, sliced
750g/1lb 10oz raw beetroot/beets,
    peeled and cut into bite-size pieces
2 tsp cumin seeds
1.25 litres/44fl oz/5½ cups vegetable
    stock, plus extra if needed
1 tsp caraway seeds
finely grated zest of 1 large orange
4–6 tbsp Greek yogurt
sea salt and freshly ground black
    pepper

Depending on the season, this vibrant-coloured beetroot/beet soup is delicious served either hot or chilled. Try it with slices of seedy rye bread for a light meal or starter to a more elaborate dinner. The soup will happily keep for up to 3 days in the refrigerator, if made in advance. Make sure you wear rubber gloves when peeling the beetroot/beets, otherwise your hands will be stained a delightful shade of pink.

⟫⟫ Heat the oil in a large heavy-based saucepan over a medium heat and cook the onion for 5 minutes, stirring regularly, until softened. Add the carrots, celery, beetroot/beet and half the cumin seeds and cook for another 2 minutes. Pour in the stock and bring to the boil, then turn the heat down slightly and simmer, part-covered, for 30 minutes, or until the vegetables are tender.

⟫⟫ Meanwhile, toast the remaining cumin and the caraway seeds in a dry, non-stick frying pan for a minute or so until they smell aromatic, then leave to one side.

⟫⟫ When the vegetables are cooked, blend the soup using a stick/immersion blender until smooth, adding a little more stock if it is too thick. Season with salt and pepper to taste and stir in half the orange zest. Stir the remaining zest into the yogurt.

⟫⟫ To serve, reheat the soup, if necessary, or chill in the refrigerator for a couple of hours. Ladle into soup bowls and top with the orange-infused yogurt and toasted spices.

Udon noodle broth

This is my go-to lunch when I'm looking for something warm and filling. A jar of dark brown rice miso paste, with its intense umami flavour, is a must for me. Don't just reserve it for Asian dishes, though – a spoonful makes an instant savoury, rich stock for all kinds of marinades, broths, soups and stews. To retain its nutritional value, try not to overheat it by boiling but instead simply warm it through before serving. This broth is one of those dishes that's readily adaptable and there are a few easy suggestions below to inspire you.

➢➢➢ Pour 1 litre/35fl oz/4⅓ cups just-boiled water into a large saucepan and place over a medium heat to keep it warm. Stir in the miso, soy and sesame oil until combined, then add the noodles and heat through briefly to separate the strands.

➢➢➢ Divide the spring onions/scallions, carrots, Chinese leaves and ginger among four large shallow bowls and ladle the noodle broth over the top, then finish with a sprinkling of nori and chilli/hot pepper flakes.

PART-TIME VARIATIONS

➢➢➢ Prawn/shrimp and bonito noodle broth

Add 300g/10½oz cooked large peeled prawns/shrimp to the serving bowls with the vegetables before pouring the hot miso noodle broth over the top. Sprinkle with bonito flakes before serving.

➢➢➢ Pork, beef or chicken noodle broth

Add shredded leftover roast pork, chicken or beef to the serving bowls just before pouring in the hot miso noodle broth. Sprinkle with chopped coriander/cilantro leaves.

SERVES ➢➢➢ 4
Preparation time ➢ 10 minutes
Cooking time ➢ 5 minutes

6 heaped tbsp brown rice miso paste
2 tbsp soy sauce
1 tbsp sesame oil
800g/1lb 12oz cooked udon noodles
6 spring onions/scallions, diagonally
    sliced
2 carrots, sliced into matchsticks
2 handfuls of shredded Chinese leaves
2cm/¾in piece of fresh root ginger,
    peeled and finely chopped
nori flakes and dried chilli/hot pepper
    flakes, to serve

Sour cherry, red quinoa AND spiced almond salad

SERVES >>> 4

Preparation time > 20 minutes,
plus 15 minutes soaking

Cooking time > 15 minutes

60g/2¼oz/scant ½ cup blanched
 almonds
½ tsp sea salt
2 tsp harissa paste
100g/3½oz/½ cup red quinoa
 (or white or black)
8 large handfuls of mixed red and
 green salad leaves
1 small red onion, halved and
 thinly sliced
2 large handfuls of mint leaves, torn
2 large handfuls of flat-leaf parsley
 leaves, torn
125g/4¼oz/scant 1 cup dried sour
 cherries or cranberries
200g/7oz firm goats' cheese, crumbled

>>> **Lemon and cumin dressing**
finely grated zest and juice of 1 large
 lemon
4 tbsp extra virgin olive oil
½ tsp cumin seeds
sea salt and freshly ground black
 pepper

The success of this salad is all about balance – you don't want any single ingredient to dominate, instead it should ideally be a harmony of taste, texture and colour.

>>> Soak the almonds in a bowl of water with the salt for 15 minutes until slightly softened. (This will help them take up the flavour of the harissa.) Drain and put them in a bowl with the harissa, turning to coat the nuts in the spice paste.

>>> Preheat the oven to 180°C/350°F/Gas 4.

>>> Put the quinoa in a saucepan and cover with water. Bring to the boil over a high heat, then turn the heat down and simmer for 12–15 minutes until tender. Drain and leave to one side.

>>> Meanwhile, put the nuts on a baking sheet, spread out evenly and roast for 10 minutes, turning once, until golden. Transfer to a bowl and leave to cool.

>>> Put the salad leaves into a large shallow serving bowl and top with the quinoa, red onion, herbs and sour cherries. Mix together the ingredients for the dressing and season with salt and pepper to taste. Spoon the dressing over the salad and toss until combined, then scatter the cheese and almonds over the top.

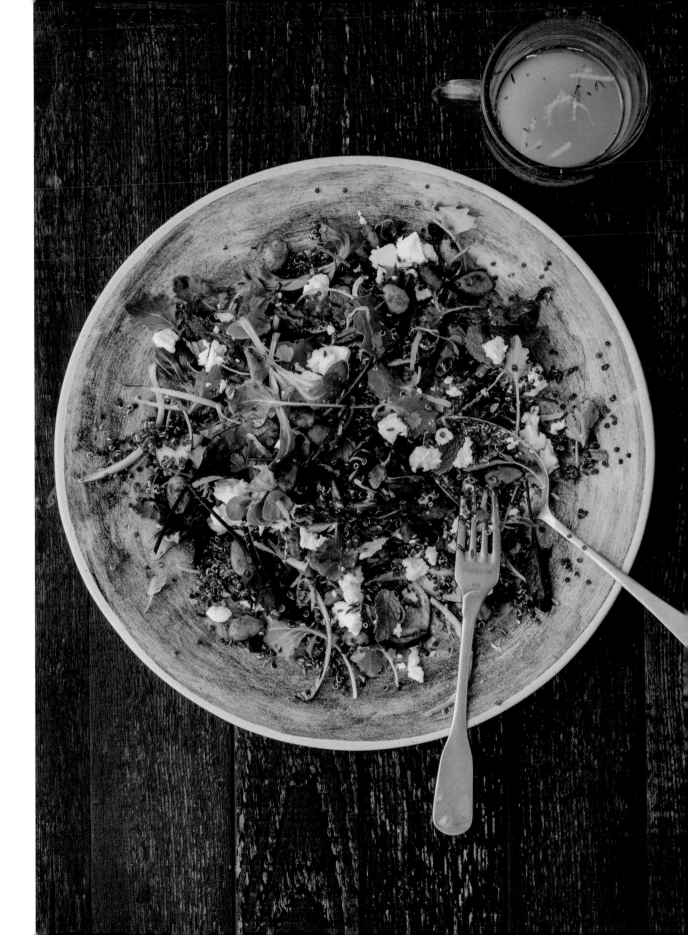

Pear, chestnut AND Gorgonzola winter salad

SERVES ⟩⟩⟩ **4**

Presentation time ⟩ 15 minutes
Cooking time ⟩ 8 minutes

40g/1½oz/2½ tbsp butter
2–3 slightly under-ripe pears
    (depending on size), peeled,
    quartered and cored
2 tbsp clear honey
165g/5¾oz/1¼ cups cooked peeled
    chestnuts, quartered
2 large red leaf Little Gem/Bibb
    lettuces or other red and green leaf
    salad, sliced
2 cooked beetroot/beets (not in
    vinegar), drained and cubed
200g/7oz Gorgonzola Piccante cheese
    or vegetarian blue cheese, rind
    removed and cut into bite-size
    pieces

⟩⟩⟩ **Lemon dressing**
juice of ½ small lemon
3 tbsp extra virgin olive oil
sea salt and freshly ground
    black pepper

A salad is an easy option that most people will enjoy as it primarily about assembling a selection of complementary ingredients – and this salad is no exception. It is full of warm flavours and textures and makes an excellent starter to a festive meal or a light meal in its own right with crusty bread. For strict vegetarians, you will need to use a vegetarian cheese as Gorgonzola uses rennet in its production. However, I do like the creamy Gorgonzola Piccante, which has a more punchy flavour than the younger and milder Gorgonzola dolce. Non-veggies could also use fresh Italian sausage instead of the cheese.

⟩⟩⟩ Mix together the ingredients for the dressing, season with salt and pepper to taste and leave to one side.

⟩⟩⟩ Melt three-quarters of the butter in a large non-stick frying pan over a medium heat. Cut each wedge of pear lengthways into two or three slices, depending on their size, and add to the pan. Cook the pears for 2 minutes on each side until starting to brown and soften.

⟩⟩⟩ Add the honey and carefully turn the pears in the glaze until glossy. Remove from the pan with a slotted spoon and add the remaining butter. When melted, add the chestnuts and cook for 2 minutes, spooning the butter mixture over them until they are warmed through and glossy. Remove the pan from the heat.

⟩⟩⟩ Divide the salad leaves between four serving plates and top with the pears, chestnuts, beetroot/beets and Gorgonzola. Spoon the dressing over the salad before serving.

PART-TIME VARIATION
⟩⟩⟩ Pear, sausage and chestnut salad

Instead of the Gorgonzola, squeeze the filling from **4–6 fresh Italian sausages** out of their skins in large bite-size chunks. Heat **1 tbsp olive oil** and fry the sausagemeat until golden and cooked through. Serve on top of the salad with the pears, chestnuts and beetroot/beets.

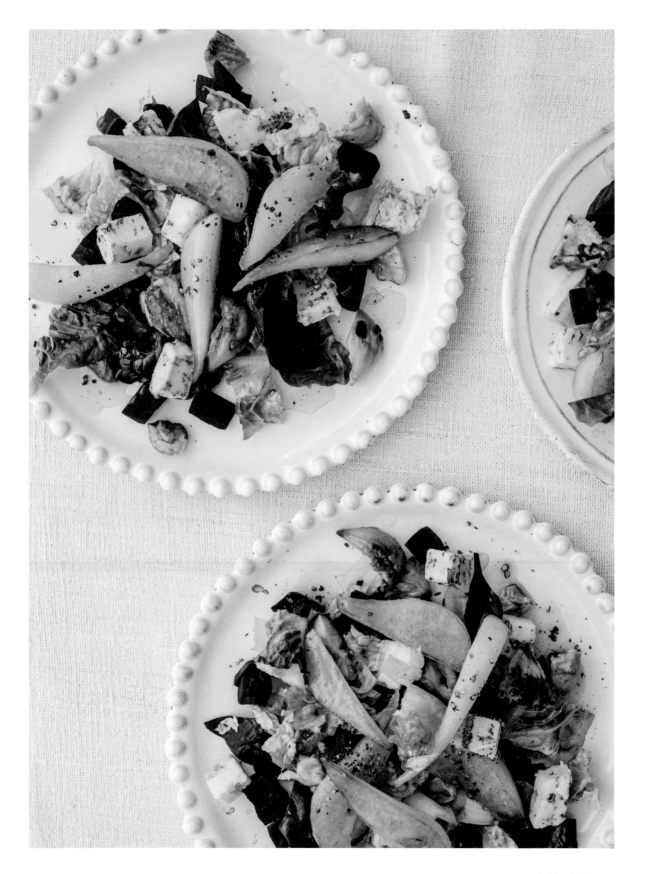

Asparagus AND Parmesan panzanella

SERVES ⟩⟩⟩ **4**

Preparation time ⟩ 15 minutes,
plus standing

Cooking time ⟩ 12 minutes

500g/1lb 2oz vine-ripened tomatoes,
  chopped into bite-size chunks

1 garlic clove, peeled and halved

2 thick slices of stale country-style
  bread, torn into bite-size chunks

2 tbsp white wine vinegar

1 orange pepper

½ red onion, diced

3 tbsp nonpareil capers, rinsed and
  patted dry

2 large handfuls of basil leaves

5 tbsp extra virgin olive oil, plus extra
  for brushing

20 asparagus spears, stalks trimmed

55g/2oz Parmesan cheese, pared into
  large shavings

sea salt and freshly ground black
  pepper

A great way of using up stale bread, this classic Italian peasant salad is vamped up with the addition of asparagus and shavings of Parmesan. The bread should have an airy crumb so it can absorb the flavours of the other ingredients – don't attempt to use it when too fresh as it will become soggy.

⟩⟩⟩ Put the tomatoes in a sieve/fine-mesh strainer suspended over a bowl, sprinkle with a little salt and crush the tomatoes slightly with the back of a fork. Leave the tomato juices to drain into the bowl.

⟩⟩⟩ Meanwhile, rub the inside of a large serving bowl with the cut side of the garlic. Add the bread and pour in the vinegar and 1 tablespoon water. Turn the bread until coated in the vinegar mixture, then leave to one side.

⟩⟩⟩ Hold the the orange pepper using tongs and carefully blacken over the flames of a hob/stovetop ring or under a hot grill/broiler, turning it occasionally, until charred all over. It will take about 8 minutes. Put the pepper in a bowl, cover with cling film/plastic wrap and leave for 5 minutes to make the skin easier to peel away.

⟩⟩⟩ Meanwhile, put the onion, capers, basil, tomatoes and their juices in the bowl with the bread. Rub the blackened skin off the pepper, cut in half, remove the seeds and chop the flesh into bite-size chunks, the same size as the tomatoes and bread, and add to the bowl. Pour the oil into the bowl and season the salad to taste with salt and pepper. Leave to stand for at least 15 minutes at room temperature to allow the flavours to mingle.

⟩⟩⟩ Heat a griddle/grill pan over a high heat. Brush the asparagus with a little oil and griddle/grill for 3–4 minutes, turning occasionally, until tender and blackened in places. Divide the panzanella among shallow serving bowls, then top with the asparagus and the Parmesan shavings.

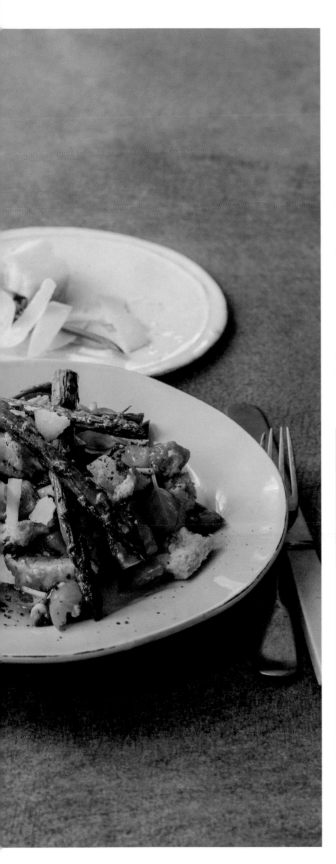

PART-TIME VARIATION

»»» Chicken panzanella

Put **4 boneless, skinless chicken breasts** between two large sheets of cling film/plastic wrap and flatten with a meat mallet or the end of a rolling pin until about 1.5cm/⅝in thick. Mix together **2 tbsp olive oil** with **2 tsp dried oregano** and **1 tsp paprika** in a large dish. Season with salt and pepper and add the chicken. Marinate, covered, in the refrigerator for 30 minutes, or longer if possible. Heat a griddle/grill pan over a high heat, then add the chicken and cook in batches for 5 minutes, turning once, until cooked through. Slice and serve on top of the salad instead of the asparagus and Parmesan.

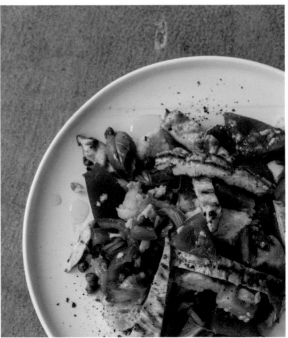

CHUTNEYS, DIPS & SALSAS

Enliven and add extra interest to a whole range of dishes, from curries and salads to snacks and soups, with this eclectic collection of chutneys, dips and salsas. All are a doddle to make and require little or no cooking.

Both the Tamarind and Date Chutney and Sweet Chilli Onion Jam are much more than just condiments and work well as part of a marinade or glaze as well as adding a touch of sweetness to tagines, stews and sauces. But if you're looking for an instant boost of flavour then the salsas are perfect. Fresh salsas are ideal when you don't feel like making a sauce but need to add a touch of moisture, colour and texture to a dish with the minimum of effort.

Dukkah is a favourite Egyptian spice and nut mix-cum-dip and is equally versatile. Use it to add flavour and texture sprinkled over warm pitta bread, soups or salads, or stir into olive oil to make a dip.

»»» Jalapeño tomato salsa

Quarter 6 vine-ripened tomatoes, scoop out the seeds, then dice the flesh. Put in a bowl and stir in 1 small diced red onion, 2 tbsp chopped pickled jalapeño chillies, 1 handful of chopped coriander/cilantro leaves and the juice of 1 lime. Season with salt and pepper before serving at room temperature.

»»» Avocado salsa

Mix the diced flesh from 1 large avocado with the juice of 1 small lime, 1 finely chopped spring onion/scallion and 2 tbsp chopped coriander/cilantro or basil leaves. Season with salt and pepper to taste and serve at room temperature.

»»» Tamarind and date chutney

Chop a **70g/2½oz block of tamarind** into pieces, discarding any seeds, and place in a saucepan with **85g/3oz/½ cup dried chopped dates, 60g/2¼oz/⅓ cup light muscovado sugar** and **250ml/9fl oz/generous 1 cup water**. Stir and bring to the boil, then turn the heat down to low and simmer for 20 minutes, part-covered, until reduced and thickened to the consistency of jam. Stir the chutney occasionally to prevent it sticking to the bottom of the pan. Press through a sieve/fine-mesh strainer to remove any seeds and fibres. Stir **1 tsp ground ginger** and **1 tbsp lime juice** into the mixture to make a thick chutney.

»»» Sweet chilli onion jam

Heat **4 tbsp olive oil** in a saucepan over a medium-low heat. Add **3 finely chopped onions** and cook gently for 20 minutes, part-covered and stirring often, until soft.

Add **3 chopped garlic cloves** and **2 medium deseeded and chopped red chillies**. Cook for another minute, then stir in **2 tbsp soft light brown sugar** and simmer over a low heat, stirring occasionally, for 8–10 minutes until reduced to a jam-like consistency. Leave chunky or use a stick/immersion blender to blend to a thick, fairly smooth jam. Leave to cool.

»»» Dukkah dip

Put **2 tbsp each of toasted coriander seeds, cumin seeds, sunflower seeds, pumpkin seeds** and **sesame seeds** (see method on page 71) in a food processor and add **40g/1½oz/⅓ cup each toasted hazelnuts** and **pistachios** (see method on page 22). Stir in **¼–½ tsp dried chilli/hot pepper flakes**, depending on taste, salt and pepper and process to a coarse, crumbly mixture – you don't want it to be too finely chopped. Transfer to a bowl and stir in enough **extra virgin olive oil** to make a dip. Store in an airtight container in the refrigerator for up to 2 weeks.

Chana crispies
WITH mango raita

SERVES ⟩⟩⟩ 4
Preparation time ⟩ 15 minutes
Cooking time ⟩ 8 minutes

400g/14oz can chickpeas, drained
1 large carrot, grated
1 red chilli, deseeded and finely
   chopped
1cm/½in piece of fresh root ginger,
   peeled and finely chopped
1 heaped tsp coriander seeds, crushed
1 heaped tsp cumin seeds, crushed
1 tsp garam masala
1 tbsp gram/chickpea/besan flour or
   plain/all-purpose flour
1 large egg, lightly beaten
sunflower oil, for frying

⟩⟩⟩ **Mango raita**
1 small mango, peeled, pitted and diced
200g/7oz/scant 1 cup plain yogurt
1 small garlic clove, crushed
juice of ½ lime
2 tbsp chopped coriander/cilantro
   leaves, plus extra to serve
sea salt and freshly ground black
   pepper

These crisp little chickpea fritters are flavoured with Indian spices and come with a fruity mango yogurt dip. Serve with a sliced cucumber, fennel and red onion salad and warm naan bread for a light meal.

⟩⟩⟩ Mix together the ingredients for the mango raita and leave to one side.

⟩⟩⟩ Put the chickpeas in a mixing bowl and roughly crush using a potato masher. Stir in the carrot, chilli, ginger, coriander, cumin, garam masala, flour and egg. Season with salt and pepper and mix everything together until combined.

⟩⟩⟩ Heat enough oil to coat the base of a large non-stick frying pan over a medium heat. Add 1 heaped dessertspoon of the chickpea mixture per fritter, flattening the tops slightly so the edges are slightly uneven. Cook in batches for 2–3 minutes on each side until golden. Drain on paper towels and keep warm in a low oven until all the mixture is used (it makes about 16 fritters in total). Serve with the mango raita with extra fresh coriander/cilantro sprinkled over the top, if you like.

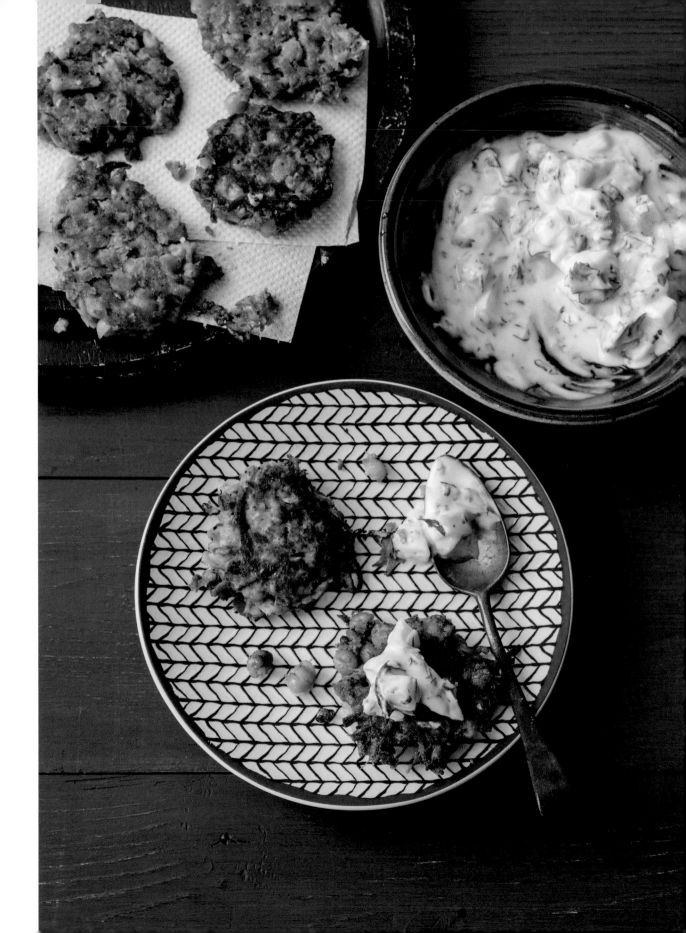

Courgette, mint
AND feta fritters

SERVES ⟩⟩⟩ **4**

Preparation time ⟩ 15 minutes
Cooking time ⟩ 20 minutes

400g/14oz courgettes/zucchini,
    coarsely grated
60g/2¼oz/½ cup plain/all-purpose
    flour
2 large eggs, lightly beaten
1 tbsp milk
200g/7oz feta cheese, patted dry
    and coarsely grated
olive oil, for frying
sea salt and freshly ground black
    pepper
2 tbsp roughly chopped unsalted
    pistachios (optional), to serve

⟩⟩⟩ **Mint yogurt sauce**

3 large handfuls of chopped
    mint leaves
250g/9oz/heaped 1 cup thick
    plain yogurt
1 small garlic clove, crushed
juice of 1 small lemon

With their flecks of green from the courgette/zucchini and mint, these good-looking feta fritters make a summery light meal served with a simple tomato salad and warm flatbreads. The mint yogurt sauce makes a fresh, herby accompaniment, or the Sweet Chilli Onion Jam (see page 67) is another good option. A sprinkling of chopped unsalted pistachios adds a contrast of texture and a pleasant crunch, but isn't essential.

⟩⟩⟩ To make the mint yogurt sauce, mix together 2 handfuls of the mint with the rest of the ingredients in a bowl. Season with salt and leave to one side.

⟩⟩⟩ Squeeze the grated courgettes/zucchini in a clean dish towel to remove any excess water, then tip them into a large mixing bowl. Stir in the flour, eggs, milk, feta and the remaining handful of mint. Season with salt and pepper, going easy on the salt as the feta is already quite salty, and stir until combined.

⟩⟩⟩ Heat enough oil to coat the base of a large non-stick frying pan over a medium heat. Add 2 tablespoons of the courgette/zucchini mixture per fritter and cook in batches for 2–3 minutes on each side until golden. Drain on paper towels and keep warm in a low oven until all the mixture is used (it makes about 12 fritters in total). Serve with the mint yogurt sauce, sprinkled with pistachios, if you like.

Mung bean humous <u>WITH</u> sesame pitta crisps

Don't be turned off by the worthy-sounding title… mung beans make a surprisingly creamy humous. Plus a bag of beans is economical to buy and their relatively short cooking time (compared with other dried beans) means that you can have a bowl of freshly made humous and pitta crisps for dunking in well under an hour.

⟩⟩⟩ Put the mung beans in a saucepan, cover with plenty of water and bring to the boil over a high heat. Reduce the heat slightly and cook on a rolling boil, part-covered, for 25 minutes, or until tender.

⟩⟩⟩ Meanwhile, make the sesame pitta crisps. Preheat the oven to 200°C/400°/Gas 6. Toast the sesame seeds in a hot dry frying pan until golden, shaking the pan occasionally so they don't boil. Brush each half of the pitta with oil. Place on baking sheets and bake for 10 minutes, or until crisp and golden. As soon as the pittas come out of the oven, brush with a little extra oil and sprinkle with the toasted sesame seeds. Leave to one side.

⟩⟩⟩ Drain the mung beans and tip them into a food processor. Add the tahini, garlic, lemon juice, olive oil and 1 tablespoon water and blend until light, smooth and creamy, adding a little more water if needed and stirring occasionally to help everything on its way.

⟩⟩⟩ Spoon the humous into a bowl and season to taste. Drizzle extra olive oil over the top before serving with the sesame pitta crisps.

SERVES ⟩⟩⟩ **4–6**
Preparation time ⟩ 15 minutes
Cooking time ⟩ 25 minutes

100g/3½oz/heaped ½ cup dried
    mung beans, rinsed
3 tbsp tahini
1 large garlic clove, crushed
juice of 1 large lemon
1 tbsp extra virgin olive oil, plus
    extra for drizzling
sea salt and freshly ground black
    pepper

⟩⟩⟩ **Sesame pitta crisps**
1 handful of sesame seeds, for
    sprinkling
4 pitta breads, split in half lengthways
    and opened out
olive oil, for brushing

Cauli cheese rarebits

SERVES ››› **4**

Preparation time › 10 minutes
Cooking time › 10 minutes

1 cauliflower, leaves removed
4 slices of country-style bread
    (optional)
1½ tbsp butter
1 tbsp plain/all-purpose flour
125ml/4fl oz/½ cup beer, light ale
    or dry cider
1 egg yolk
2 tsp English mustard
a pinch of cayenne pepper
150g/5½oz/1½ cups grated mature
    Cheddar cheese
freshly ground black pepper
tomato and chive salad, to serve

This recipe combines two British favourites – cauliflower cheese and Welsh rarebit – in a single dish. Cauliflower is an amazing vegetable and there is so much you can do with it: try puréeing steamed cauli with a combination of stock and cream to make a delicious sauce; grating it raw into grain-size pieces and tossing in a garlicky vinaigrette dressing; or marinating in olive oil and spices and roasting until golden. Don't discard the green outer leaves, either, as they can be chopped into stir-fries, soups and salads or tossed in oil and roasted whole – they taste similar to kale.

››› The easiest way to prepare the caulilflower is to slice it in half vertically through the middle and then cut 1.5cm/⅝in thick slices from the mid cross-section to make 'steaks'. Steam the cauliflower for 2 minutes until just starting to soften. Remove from the steamer and leave to one side, taking care as the steaks are quite fragile and you want to keep the florets intact.

››› Meanwhile, if you are serving the dish on toast, preheat the grill/broiler to high. Lightly toast both sides of each slice of bread.

››› To make the cheese rarebit topping, melt the butter in a small saucepan over a low heat, then stir in the flour. Cook for 1 minute, stirring constantly. Slowly add the beer, stirring to make a smooth sauce. Stir in the egg yolk, mustard, cayenne and Cheddar and continue to cook until you have a thick, smooth sauce, stirring continuously.

››› Turn the grill/broiler to medium and line a roasting pan with foil. Spread the cheese sauce thickly on top of each cauliflower steak and grill/broil for 3–5 minutes until the sauce starts to bubble and turn golden. Place the cauliflower steaks on top of the toasts, if using, season with pepper and serve with a tomato and chive salad (you could grill the tomatoes briefly to make a warm salad).

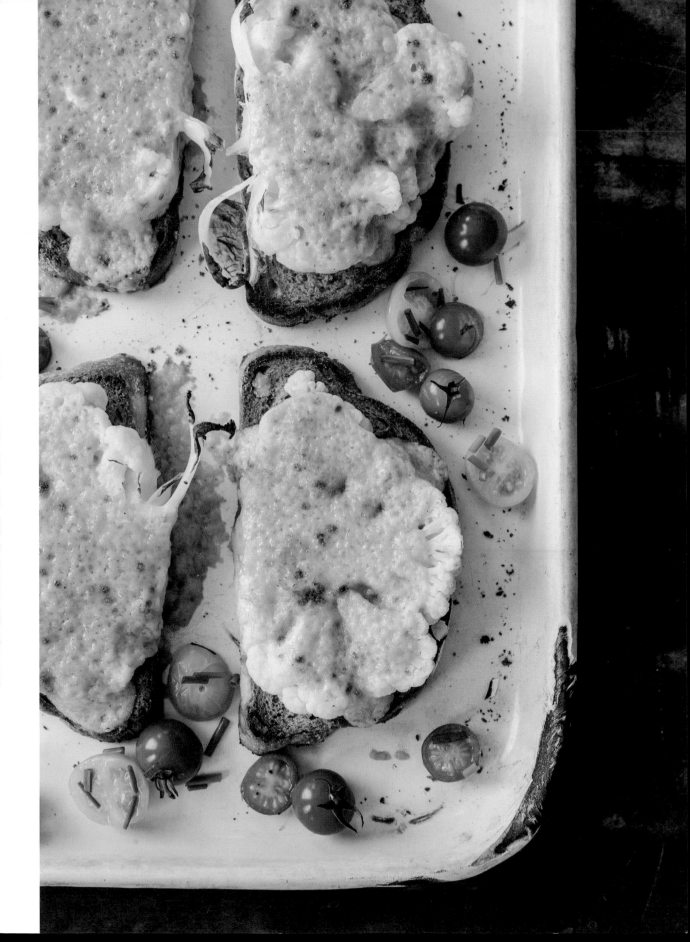

Labneh

Preparation time 〉 10 minutes,
plus draining overnight

500g/1lb 2oz/2 heaped cups Greek
   yogurt or thick plain yogurt
1½ tsp sea salt
flatbreads, crackers, figs and rocket/
   arugula salad, to serve

〉〉〉 **Walnut topping**
2 handfuls of walnuts, toasted (see
   method on page 22) and roughly
   chopped
seeds (arils) from ¼ pomegranate
a few mint sprigs, leaves torn
1–2 tbsp clear honey, such as chestnut
1 tbsp extra virgin olive oil

Try your hand at cheesemaking with this simple
Middle Eastern drained yogurt cheese, which is
similar in consistency to a thick cream cheese or
curd cheese and has a mild, slightly acidic flavour.
It's also incredibly versatile and can be adapted to
suit both sweet and savoury dishes – see Lebanese
Lentils with Labneh Balls on page 172 – and is great
with a range of accompaniments, from fresh figs and
nuts to anchovies and charcuterie. Perfect for
a sharing platter with friends and family.

〉〉〉 Line a sieve/fine-mesh strainer with a piece of muslin
or cheesecloth large enough to hang over the sides (or use
a new J-cloth). Suspend the sieve/fine-mesh strainer over
a mixing bowl.

〉〉〉 Mix the yogurt with the salt and spoon it into the cloth-
lined sieve/fine-mesh strainer. Pull the cloth up around the
yogurt and twist the top to make a bundle. Leave the yogurt
in the refrigerator to drain for at least 12 hours, preferably
up to 24 hours – the longer you leave it, the firmer the
labneh will be. Give the bundle a gentle squeeze every
so often to encourage any whey to drain away.

〉〉〉 Remove the muslin bundle from the sieve/fine-mesh
strainer and open it to reveal a smooth ball of soft cheese.
The labneh is ready to eat. Simply place it in a serving bowl
or plate, scatter the walnuts, pomegranate seeds and mint
over the top and drizzle with honey and olive oil. Serve
with flatbreads, crackers, figs and a rocket/arugula salad.

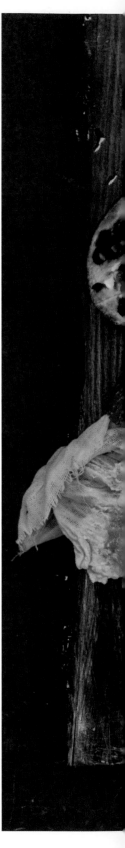

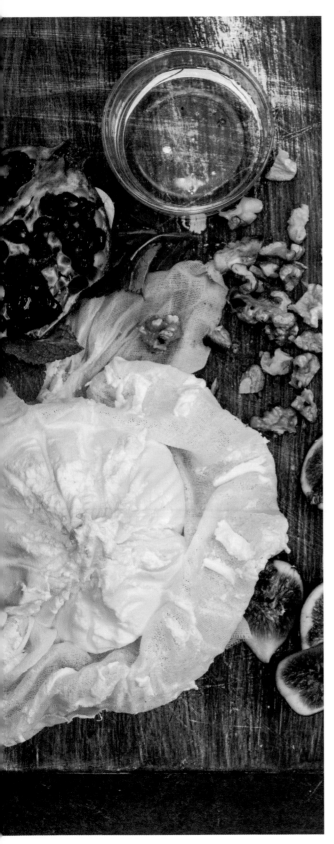

PART-TIME VARIATIONS

››› Labneh with charcuterie

Roll the labneh into balls and coat in a mixture of
fresh herbs and chilli/hot pepper flakes. Serve with
a selection of charcuterie, figs, olives and crusty bread.

››› Labneh with olives and anchovies

Top the labneh with a few spoonfuls of Olive Tapenade
(see page 36) and serve with a tomato and anchovy salad.

››› Labneh with harissa and lamb

Mash a spoonful of labneh with harissa paste and a little
olive oil and use as a stuffing for a chicken breast or spoon
on top of a chargrilled lamb fillet.

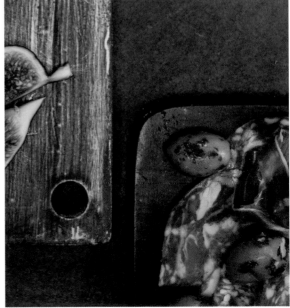

Roasted aubergine
<u>WITH</u> miso

SERVES ⟩⟩⟩ **4**

Preparation time ⟩ 10 minutes

Cooking time ⟩ 30 minutes

2 aubergines/eggplants, halved
    lengthways

2 tbsp sesame oil, plus extra for
    greasing

2 tbsp dark miso paste

2 tbsp soy sauce

2 tbsp mirin

2 tsp clear honey

1cm/½in piece of fresh root ginger,
    peeled and grated

3 spring onions/scallions, diagonally
    sliced

½ tsp shichimi togarashi or dried chilli/
    hot pepper flakes (optional)

jasmine rice and steamed pak choi/bok
    choy, to serve

When I tested this recipe, I was told that it was the best aubergine/ eggplant dish I'd ever made – praise indeed from someone who doesn't particularly like aubergine/eggplant. And what's more, it's so easy to make. Shichimi togarashi is a Japanese spice blend based on chilli, orange peel, sesame seeds, Szechuan pepper and seaweed. It's not essential here, but it does add an aromatic chilli zing to the final dish. You can find it in large supermarkets or Asian grocers.

⟩⟩⟩ Preheat the oven to 200°C/400°F/Gas 6. Score the flesh of each aubergine/ eggplant half diagonally both ways, then brush all over (skin included) with half the sesame oil. Put the aubergines/eggplants, cut-side down, in a large oiled roasting pan and roast for 20 minutes until softened.

⟩⟩⟩ Mix the remaining sesame oil with the miso paste, soy sauce, mirin, honey and ginger and brush the mixture over the cut side of each aubergine/eggplant. Return them to the oven, cut-side up, and roast for a further 8–10 minutes, or until golden. Sprinkle with spring onions/scallions and shichimi togarashi, if using, and serve with jasmine rice and steamed pak choi/bok choy.

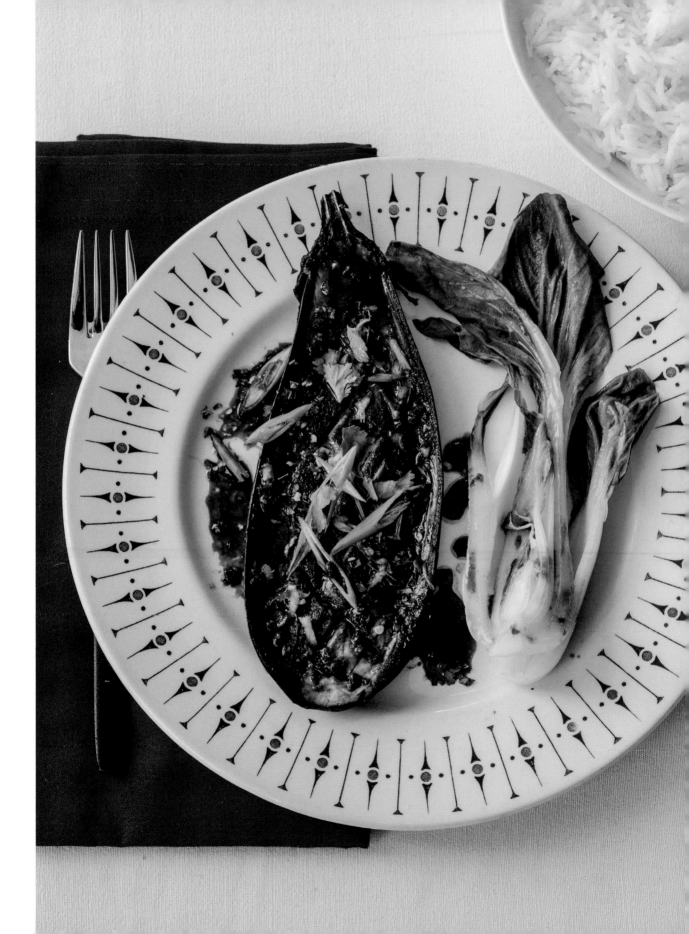

Baked sweet potato
WITH za'atar

SERVES ⟫⟫ **4 (WITH LEFTOVER ZA'ATAR)**

Preparation time ⟫ 10 minutes
Cooking time ⟫ 55 minutes

4 sweet potatoes
4 heaped tbsp crème fraîche or sour cream
1 red chilli, deseeded and finely chopped
1 handful of flaked/slivered almonds, toasted (see method on page 22)
mixed leaf salad, to serve

⟫⟫ **Za'atar**

3 tbsp thyme leaves or 1½ tbsp dried
2 tsp sumac
½ tsp sea salt
1 tbsp sesame seeds, toasted (see page 71)

A sweet potato, when baked, is the ultimate comfort food. Its soft, yielding texture and slight sweetness is countered here by the tangy crunch of the Middle Eastern spice mix, za'atar. You can buy ready-made za'atar, but it's easy to make your own and it is worth experimenting with different blends of herbs and spices. If you are unfamiliar with the spice sumac, this ground deep pinky-red berry has a slightly tart, lemony flavour and, like shop-bought za'atar, can be found in larger supermarkets, in Middle Eastern grocers or online. Keep a jar for when you want to liven up yogurt, humous, eggs, soups and salads or whatever takes your fancy.

⟫⟫ Preheat the oven to 160°C/315°F/Gas 2½. Put the thyme on a small baking sheet in the oven for 5 minutes, or until dried but still retaining its green colour.

⟫⟫ Turn the oven up to 200°C/400°F/Gas 6. Bake the sweet potatoes for 40–50 minutes, depending on their size, until tender.

⟫⟫ Meanwhile, finish making the za'atar. Crumble the thyme into a bowl and mix in the sumac, salt and sesame seeds, then leave to one side.

⟫⟫ Make a cut into the top of each potato, squeeze open slightly, then top with a spoonful of crème fraîche and scatter over the chilli, za'atar and almonds. Serve with a mixed leaf salad. (Store any leftover za'atar in an airtight container for up to 2 weeks.)

Creamy mustard <u>AND</u> spinach lentils

This simple recipe uses canned green lentils to make a quick lunch, but if time allows dried lentils don't take that much longer to cook and are more economical to buy. A crumbly goats' or sheep's cheese is scattered over the top just before serving, but this could easily be smoked bacon if you're looking for an easy-to-adapt meal. A slice of country-style bread griddled until golden and crisp then rubbed with the cut side of a clove of garlic is the perfect accompaniment.

>>> Heat the oil in a large non-stick sauté pan over a medium-low heat and cook the spinach for 2–3 minutes, turning the leaves with tongs until evenly wilted. Add the garlic, tomatoes and lentils and cook for 3 minutes, stirring regularly.

>>> Add the mustard, lemon juice and crème fraîche, season with salt and pepper and warm through for a couple of minutes, stirring until combined. Crumble over the cheese and serve with slices of griddled garlicky toast.

PART-TIME VARIATION

>>> Smoked bacon and spinach lentils

Bacon and lentils is a classic partnership. Instead of the crumbly cheese, grill/broil **6 rashers smoked streaky bacon** until crisp. Drain on paper towels, then crumble over the lentil mixture just before serving.

SERVES >>> 4

Preparation time >> 10 minutes
Cooking time >> 8 minutes

2 tbsp olive oil
175g/6oz baby leaf spinach
3 garlic cloves, finely chopped
5 vine-ripened tomatoes, deseeded
    and diced
2 × 400g/14oz cans green or brown
    lentils, drained
1 tbsp wholegrain mustard
juice of ½ large lemon
5 tbsp crème fraîche
100g/3½oz Lancashire cheese, or firm
    goats' or sheep's cheese, crumbled
sea salt and freshly ground black
    pepper
thick slices of griddled toast rubbed
    with garlic, to serve

Char sui tofu cups

SERVES 〉〉〉 **4**

Preparation time 〉 20 minutes, plus marinating
Cooking time 〉 25 minutes

6 tbsp char sui or hoisin sauce

2 tbsp sweet chilli sauce

1 tbsp soy sauce

2 tsp sesame oil

2.5cm/1in piece of fresh root ginger, peeled and finely chopped

400g/14oz block of tofu, drained well on paper towels, then cut into 1cm/½in cubes

1 tbsp sunflower oil

2 small Little Gem/Bibb lettuces, leaves separated (you need about 20 leaves)

2 spring onions/scallions, finely sliced diagonally

2 tbsp sesame seeds, toasted (see page 71)

1 red chilli, deseeded and finely chopped

For golden, crisp tofu, it's vital to drain it well to remove any excess water, which would also dilute the intensity of the marinade. Instead of the spring onion/scallion, sesame and chilli topping, you could also serve the tofu topped with Easy Kimchi (see page 165), or with noodles and stir-fried greens for a more substantial meal. Alternatively, if serving as a starter or party food, why not fill some of the lettuce parcels with the char sui duck variation.

〉〉〉 Mix together the char sui sauce, sweet chilli sauce, soy sauce, sesame oil and ginger in a large, shallow dish. Add the tofu and gently turn to coat it in the marinade, then leave to marinate for at least 1 hour.

〉〉〉 Preheat the oven to 200°C/400°F/Gas 6. Heat the sunflower oil on a large baking sheet and, when hot, add the tofu in a single layer. Roast for 25 minutes, turning once, until golden and slightly crisp. Meanwhile, warm any leftover marinade with a splash of water in a small pan.

〉〉〉 Arrange the lettuce leaves on a large serving platter and divide the tofu among them, placing it inside the 'cups'. Spoon a little of the warm marinade over each one and scatter with the spring onions/scallions, sesame seeds and chilli.

PART-TIME VARIATION

〉〉〉 Char sui duck

Although char sui pork fillet is perhaps more usual, the marinade also works with duck. Score the skin of **2 large duck breasts** and add to the marinade. Leave to marinate for 1 hour, occasionally spooning the marinade over the duck. Place the duck, skin-side down, in a cold, dry, non-stick frying pan over a medium heat for 7 minutes until golden, then turn over and brown for 1 minute. Regularly pour off any fat that accumulates in the pan.

Preheat the oven to 220°C/425°C/Gas 7, spoon more of the marinade over the duck and place, skin-side up, on a rack over a roasting pan. Roast for 15 minutes, or until the duck is cooked to your liking, then leave to rest for 5 minutes. Cut diagonally into slices and serve as instructed above in place of the tofu.

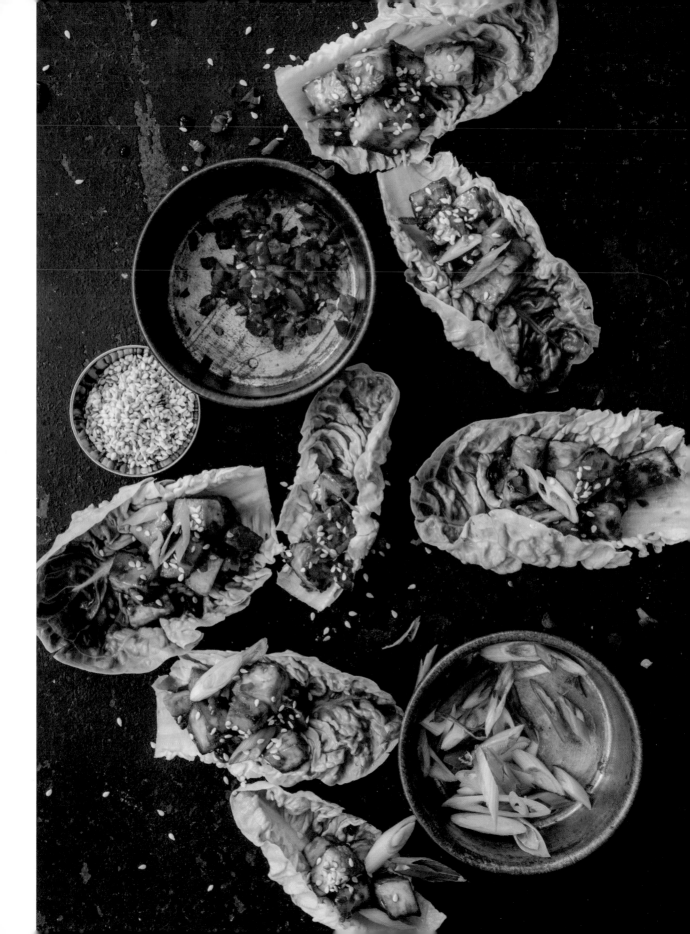

Steamed tofu IN ginger-soy dressing

SERVES ⟩⟩⟩ **4**

Preparation time ⟩ 10 minutes
Cooking time ⟩ 5 minutes

400g/14oz block of firm tofu, drained
   well on paper towels
6 tbsp Chinese rice wine or dry sherry
4 tbsp mirin
2 tbsp light soy sauce
4 tsp sesame oil
2cm/¾in piece of fresh root ginger,
   peeled and thinly sliced
1 red chilli, deseeded and sliced into
   thin strips
3 spring onions/scallions, sliced into
   thin strips
1 handful of basil leaves, preferably
   Thai, torn
brown basmati rice and steamed
   long-stem broccoli, to serve

Simplicity itself… steamed tofu is the perfect counter to the fragrant, punchy, ginger-soy dressing. Serve the tofu dish with brown basmati rice or egg noodles and steamed green vegetables for a more substantial meal. Or fish-eaters could try the version opposite, made with pollock.

⟩⟩⟩ Make a few holes in a sheet of baking paper, then use it to line a steamer basket. Place the basket over a pan or wok of gently simmering water. Add the tofu and steam for 5 minutes until warmed through and softer in texture. Remove the basket from the heat, leave to drain for a minute or so, then lift the tofu out using the paper to help and transfer to a serving plate.

⟩⟩⟩ Meanwhile, mix together the Chinese rice wine, mirin, soy sauce, sesame oil and ginger in a small pan over a high heat. Bring almost to the boil, then turn the heat down and simmer for 3 minutes until reduced slightly.

⟩⟩⟩ Spoon the sauce over the tofu and top with the chilli, spring onions/scallions and basil. Serve with rice and steamed long-stem broccoli (you can steam the broccoli at the same time as the tofu).

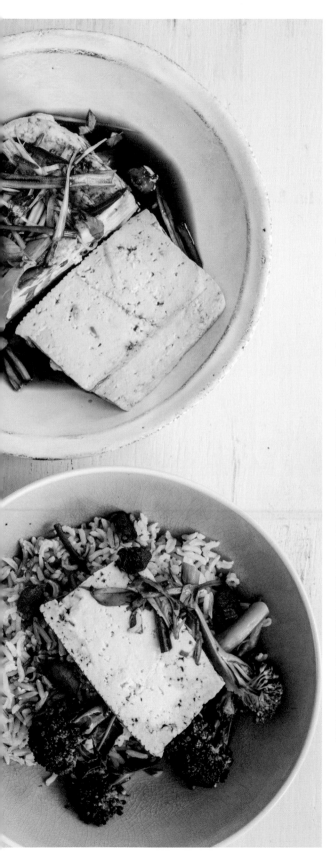

PART-TIME VARIATION
»»» Chilli and ginger pollock

Firm fillets of white fish, such as pollock, or alternatively oily fish, including salmon, trout and mackerel, work with this Chinese-inspired sauce. Put 175g/6oz pollock fillet per person on a piece of baking paper and top with the thinly sliced ginger, chilli and spring onions/scallions. Season with salt and pepper and fold the paper over to make a parcel. Steam for 5 minutes, or until cooked. Prepare the sauce as described, and spoon it over the fish. Sprinkle with basil before serving.

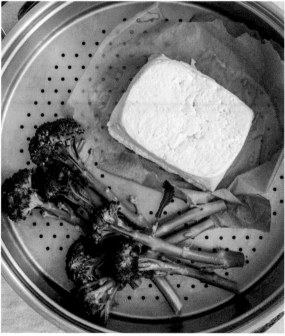

Corn flatbread pizzas

MAKES ⟩⟩⟩ **6**

Preparation time ⟩ 20 minutes, plus rising

Cooking time ⟩ 40 minutes

⟩⟩⟩ **Corn flatbreads**

1 tsp instant dried yeast

150ml/5fl oz/scant ⅔ cup lukewarm water

100g/3½oz/⅔ cup fine polenta/ cornmeal

200g/7oz/1½ cups strong bread flour, plus extra for dusting

1 tsp sea salt

2 tsp extra virgin olive oil, plus extra for greasing and to serve

2 tbsp plain yogurt

⟩⟩⟩ **To serve**

1 recipe quantity Jalapeño Tomato Salsa (see page 66)

250g/9oz mozzarella cheese, patted dry and torn into pieces

6 handfuls of rocket/arugula leaves

4 tbsp Dukkah Dip, omitting the olive oil (see page 67)

This twist on the Italian classic *pizza bianca* features a corn flatbread base with a vegetarian topping of tomato salsa, rocket/arugula, mozzarella and a sprinkling of the North African nut and spice mix, dukkah. There is also the option of spiced marinated lamb – why not let everyone help themselves to their favourite toppings at the table? Incidentally, the uncooked flatbread dough, or indeed the cooked breads, will keep in the freezer for up to three months, so it makes sense to make extra for next time.

⟩⟩⟩ Mix the yeast with a little of the water and leave until slightly frothy. Mix together the polenta/cornmeal, flour and salt in a large mixing bowl and make a well in the middle. Pour in the yeasted water, the remaining water, the olive oil and yogurt, then gradually draw the dry ingredients into the wet using a fork and then your fingers to make a ball of dough. Knead on a lightly floured work surface for 10 minutes until smooth and elastic. Put the dough into a lightly oiled mixing bowl, cover with cling film/plastic wrap and leave in a warm place to rise for 1½ hours or until doubled in size.

⟩⟩⟩ Tip the dough out onto a lightly floured work surface and divide into 6 balls, then roll into large, thin rounds. Heat a large non-stick frying pan until hot, brush with oil and cook the flatbreads, one at a time, for 2–3 minutes on each side until slightly golden and cooked through. Cover with a cloth or foil to keep warm while you cook all the flatbreads.

⟩⟩⟩ To serve, top each warm flatbread with the salsa, mozzarella, rocket/arugula and dukkah and finish with a drizzle of olive oil.

PART-TIME VARIATION

⟩⟩⟩ **Lamb flatbread pizzas**

Marinate **4 lamb steaks**, about 140g/5oz each, in 2 tsp each of coarsely crushed **coriander** and **cumin seeds** and **dried mint** combined with **4 tbsp olive oil** and a **squeeze of lemon juice**. Season with salt and pepper and marinate for up to 1 hour. Heat a griddle/grill pan or large heavy-based frying pan over a high heat and sear the lamb for 5 minutes, turning once, or until cooked to your liking. Cover and leave to rest for 5 minutes before cutting into slices and serving instead of the mozzarella.

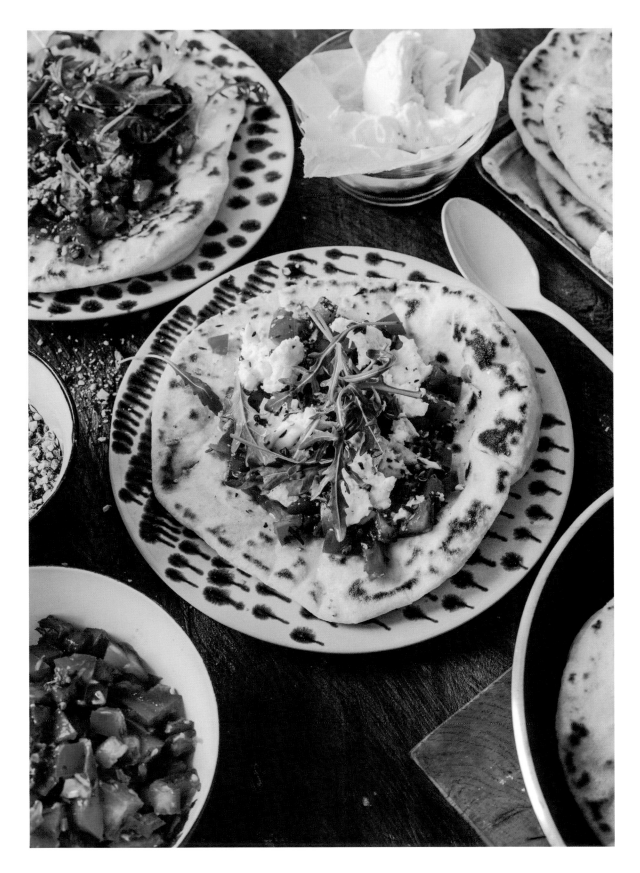

Sag aloo wraps

SERVES ⟩⟩⟩ **4**

Preparation time ⟩ 15 minutes
Cooking time ⟩ 25 minutes

2 tbsp coconut oil
550g/1lb 4oz potatoes, peeled and
    cut into 1cm/½in cubes
1 large onion, halved and thinly sliced
2 garlic cloves, chopped
2.5cm/1in piece of fresh root ginger,
    grated
1 tsp cumin seeds
1 tsp nigella seeds
1 tsp turmeric
1–2 green chillies, deseeded and
    chopped
200g/7oz spinach leaves, tough
    stalks discarded
4 chapatis, warmed, or Dosa
    (see page 188)
sea salt and freshly ground black
    pepper

⟩⟩⟩ **Mint raita**
6 tbsp plain yogurt
1 handful of chopped mint leaves
1 small garlic clove, crushed
juice of 1 lime

Equally good served at room temperature as it is warm, this spiced, dry potato and spinach curry makes a substantial filling for an Indian-style wrap. More commonly served as a side dish to curries, sag aloo would also stand up as a meal in itself with the addition of halved cherry tomatoes and chickpeas and topped with fried cashews. This dish is also a perfect way to use up any leftover cooked potatoes – just warm through with the spices and spinach.

⟩⟩⟩ Heat the oil in a large heavy-based sauté pan over a medium heat. Add the potatoes and cook, covered and stirring occasionally, for 15 minutes until tender and golden in places. Remove from the pan with a slotted spoon and leave to one side, then add the onion and cook for another 5 minutes, covered, until softened.

⟩⟩⟩ Meanwhile, mix together all the ingredients for the mint raita, using half of the lime juice.

⟩⟩⟩ Return the potatoes to the sauté pan with the garlic, ginger, all the spices and the chilli. Stir until combined, then add the spinach, the reserved lime juice and a splash of water, cover, and cook for 5 minutes, stirring occasionally, until the spinach has wilted. Season with salt and pepper to taste.

⟩⟩⟩ Meanwhile, warm the chapatis, two at a time, in a large dry frying pan. To assemble the wraps, spoon the sag aloo down one side of each chapati, top with a good spoonful of the raita, fold in the ends and then roll up. Cut in half crossways before serving. Repeat to make four wraps in total, then serve warm or at room temperature.

Mexican eggs
WITH corn chips

The Mexican chipotle – a smoked and dried jalapeño chilli – gives a distinctive smoky heat to this spiced tomato sauce. The eggs are cooked nestled in the sauce with crisp corn tortillas for dunking. If you can't find dried chipotle chillies or paste, 1 teaspoon dried chilli/hot pepper flakes or 1 teaspoon hot smoked paprika are worthy alternatives. Serve with a simple, crisp green leaf salad.

⟩⟩⟩ Pour enough just-boiled water over the chipotle chilli to cover and leave to soften for 20 minutes.

⟩⟩⟩ Heat 2 tablespoons of the oil in a large deep sauté pan over a medium heat and fry the onion for 8 minutes, stirring regularly, until softened. Drain the chipotle, discarding the soaking water, and chop finely. (Discard the seeds if you don't want the sauce to be too hot.) Add the chilli, both peppers and garlic to the onion and cook for a further 3 minutes until softened.

⟩⟩⟩ Stir in the oregano, cumin seeds, tomatoes, ketchup and bring to the boil, then turn the heat down and simmer for 10 minutes, stirring regularly, until reduced and thickened. Season with salt and pepper to taste. Make 4 holes or dips in the tomato sauce and tip in the eggs, cover the pan and simmer for 3–4 minutes until the egg whites are set but the yolks remain runny.

⟩⟩⟩ Meanwhile, preheat the oven to 200°/400°C/Gas 6. Put the tortillas in the oven, placing them directly on the oven shelves and spread apart, for 10 minutes, or until crisp. Brush with the remaining oil, sprinkle with cumin seeds, leave to cool, then break into large pieces. Serve the Mexican eggs topped with coriander/cilantro and the corn chips by the side.

SERVES ⟩⟩⟩ **4**

Preparation time ⟩ 20 minutes, plus soaking
Cooking time ⟩ 25 minutes

1 dried chipotle chilli or 1 tbsp chipotle paste
3 tbsp olive oil
1 large onion, finely chopped
1 red pepper, deseeded and chopped
1 green pepper, deseeded and chopped
1 large garlic clove, finely chopped
1 tsp dried oregano
1 tsp cumin seeds, plus extra for sprinkling
2 x 400g/14oz cans chopped tomatoes
1 tbsp tomato ketchup
4 large eggs
4 soft corn tortillas
sea salt and freshly ground black pepper
1 handful of coriander/cilantro leaves, to serve

PART-TIME VARIATION
⟩⟩⟩ Mexican eggs with prawns/shrimp

Chorizo is an obvious alternative, or addition, to the eggs but prawns/shrimps also work well with the smoky heat of the sauce. Stir in **350g/12oz raw, peeled large prawns/jumbo shrimp** into the sauce and cook, stirring occasionally, for 3 minutes until pink and cooked through, then stir in the eggs. Serve topped with coriander/cilantro and with crusty bread and a green salad.

Coddled eggs WITH kohlrabi remoulade

SERVES ⟫⟫ **4**

Preparation time ⟫ 15 minutes

Cooking time ⟫ 12 minutes

butter, for greasing

8 eggs

4–8 slices of toasted rye bread,
depending on size

2 tbsp snipped chives

⟫⟫ Kohlrabi remoulade

1 kohlrabi or celeriac, peeled and cut
into thin matchsticks

4 tbsp mayonnaise

1 heaped tsp Dijon mustard

5 small gherkins, drained and sliced

2–3 tbsp lemon juice

1 handful of chopped parsley leaves

sea salt and freshly ground black
pepper

Coddling is a traditional and gentle method of steaming eggs in a water bath, usually in a coddler, which resembles a small ceramic pot with a lid. As I don't own a coddler, I used a deep ramekin instead with a piece of cling film/plastic wrap in place of a lid and the result was just as good. The eggs come with remoulade, classically a winter salad made with celeriac, but this summer alternative is made with crisp shreds of kohlrabi, or you could use radish, cucumber, turnip or mooli. The remoulade goes equally well with fresh mackerel for your non-vegetarian family or guests.

⟫⟫ Mix together all the ingredients for the remoulade in a bowl, season with salt and pepper, and leave to one side until ready to serve.

⟫⟫ Meanwhile, pour sufficient water to come halfway up the sides of 4 large, deep ramekins into a sauté pan with a lid. Bring the water to the boil. Liberally grease the ramekins with butter and crack two eggs into each one. Cover tightly with cling film/plastic wrap and carefully lower the ramekins into the pan. Turn the heat to a gentle boil and cook the eggs for 4 minutes, then turn the heat down to its lowest setting and let the eggs cook for another 7 minutes, or until the white is set but the yolks remain runny.

⟫⟫ Spoon the remoulade on top of the slices of rye toast. Run a knife around the inside edge of the ramekins to loosen the eggs then turn them out on top of the remoulade. Season and sprinkle with chives before serving.

PART-TIME VARIATION

⟫⟫ Mackerel with remoulade on rye

Season **4 large fresh mackerel fillets** and melt **1 ½ tbsp butter** in a large non-stick frying pan over a medium heat. Place the mackerel in the pan, skin-side down, and cook for 2–3 minutes until crisp, then turn over and cook for another 2 minutes, or until cooked. Squeeze **a little lemon juice** over the mackerel and serve on the remoulade-topped rye toast instead of the coddled eggs.

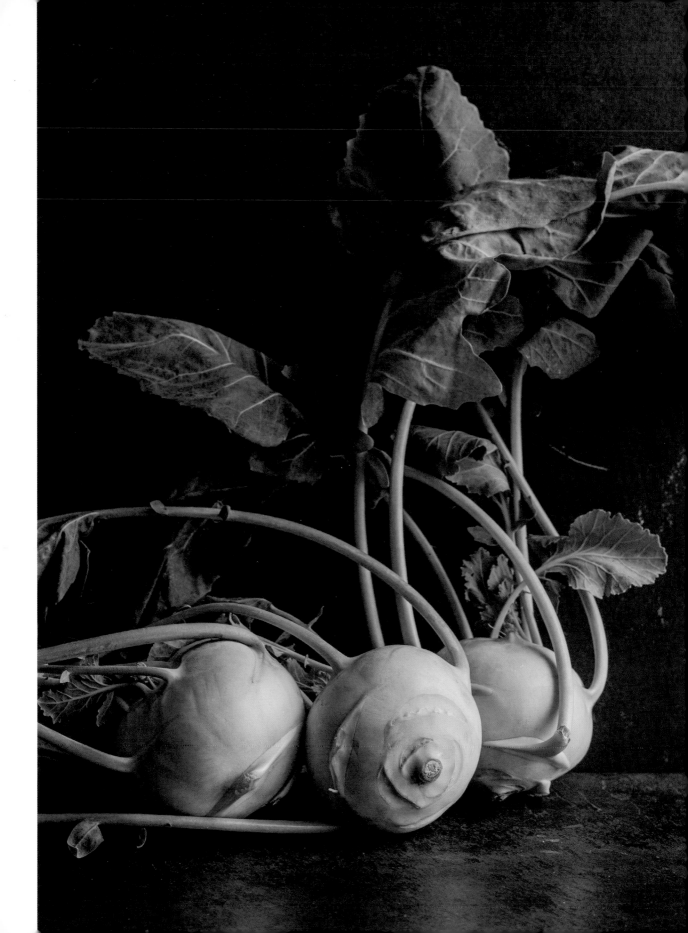

Thai vegetable omelette

SERVES ⟩⟩⟩ **2**

Preparation time ⟩ 15 minutes
Cooking time ⟩ 10 minutes

4 tsp coconut oil
1 carrot, cut into thin strips
½ red pepper, deseeded and sliced
    into thin strips
3 spring onions/scallions, thinly
    sliced diagonally
125g/4½oz hispi cabbage, shredded
1cm/½in piece of fresh root ginger,
    peeled and cut into thin strips
1 large garlic clove, thinly sliced
1 tbsp light soy sauce
1 tsp sesame oil
4 large eggs, lightly beaten
1 handful of basil leaves, preferably Thai
freshly ground black pepper
warm naan bread, to serve

Thai, or holy, basil is a fragrant combination of aniseed crossed with regular basil and is unmistakably Asian in flavour. It can be found in some large supermarkets or more usually Asian grocers and it's really worth trying for its distinctive taste. What's more, in Ayurvedic medicine holy basil is reputed to relieve stress and lift the spirit (hence its name). You could even serve this Thai-style omelette with an aromatic infusion of holy basil, lemongrass and ginger.

⟩⟩⟩ Melt half the coconut oil in a large non-stick frying pan over a high heat and stir-fry the carrot, red pepper, spring onions/scallions and cabbage for 3 minutes until tender.

⟩⟩⟩ Turn the heat down to medium, add the ginger and garlic and stir-fry for another minute. Remove from the heat and add 1 teaspoon of the soy sauce and the sesame oil. Transfer the vegetables to a bowl, cover, and keep them warm while you cook the omelettes. Wipe the frying pan clean.

⟩⟩⟩ Lightly beat two of the eggs with 1 teaspoon of the soy sauce and season with pepper. Heat 1 teaspoon of the coconut oil in the frying pan, add the egg and tilt the pan to coat the base. Cook for a few minutes, drawing any of the cooked egg to the middle of the pan, until just set.

⟩⟩⟩ Slide the omelette onto a plate and top one half with half of the stir-fried vegetables. Top with half the basil and fold the omelette over to encase the vegetables. Repeat to make a second omelette. Serve straight away with warm naan bread.

PART-TIME VARIATION
⟩⟩⟩ Thai chicken omelette

Slice 2 skinless, boneless chicken breasts, about 175g/6oz each, into thin strips and marinate in 1 tbsp soy sauce and 1 tbsp fish sauce for 30 minutes. Stir-fry for 2 minutes before adding the vegetables, as described above.

Spinach AND broad bean frittata

A dish full of the flavours of summer. The key to a successful frittata is to get the balance of filling to egg just right, as an overly eggy one can, quite frankly, be a little dull. If fresh broad/fava beans are out of season, opt for frozen, which make a more than adequate substitute. Frittatas are also best cooked gently, otherwise they are prone to turn rubbery.

⟩⟩⟩ Steam the broad/fava beans for 2 minutes, or until tender, then refresh under cold running water. Gently squeeze the beans out of their grey outer skin to reveal a bright green inner bean. Mix the beans with the spinach, spring onions/scallions and mint.

⟩⟩⟩ Preheat the grill/broiler to medium. Mix together the eggs and Parmesan and season with salt and pepper. Pour into the vegetable mixture and stir until everything is mixed together.

⟩⟩⟩ Melt the butter in a medium non-stick, ovenproof frying pan over a medium-low heat. Pour in the egg mixture and cook for 5 minutes, or until the base of the frittata is light golden and set, then place the pan under the grill/broiler and cook for another 5–8 minutes, or until just set. Remove from the grill/broiler, cover and leave to stand for a couple of minutes before cutting into wedges and serving with crusty bread and salad.

SERVES ⟩⟩⟩ **4–6**

Preparation time ⟩ 15 minutes
Cooking time ⟩ 15 minutes

250g/9oz/2 cups shelled broad/fava
    beans, fresh or frozen
125g/4½oz baby leaf spinach, finely
    chopped
5 spring onions/scallions, finely
    chopped
1 large handful of chopped mint leaves
7 eggs, lightly beaten
30g/1oz/scant ½ cup finely grated
    Parmesan cheese
1½ tbsp butter
sea salt and freshly ground black
    pepper
crusty bread and mixed salad,
    to serve

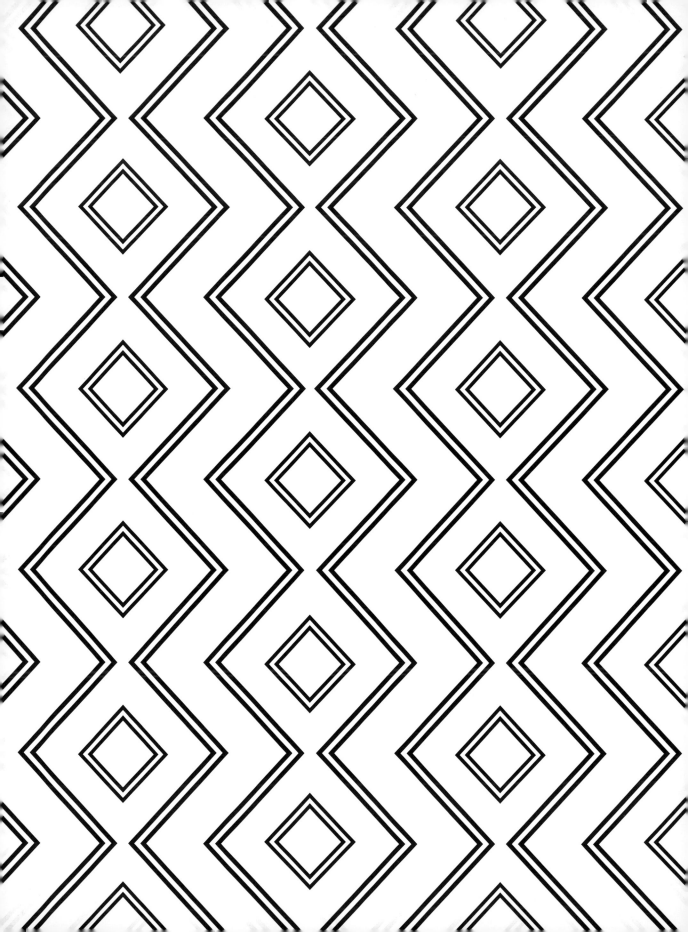

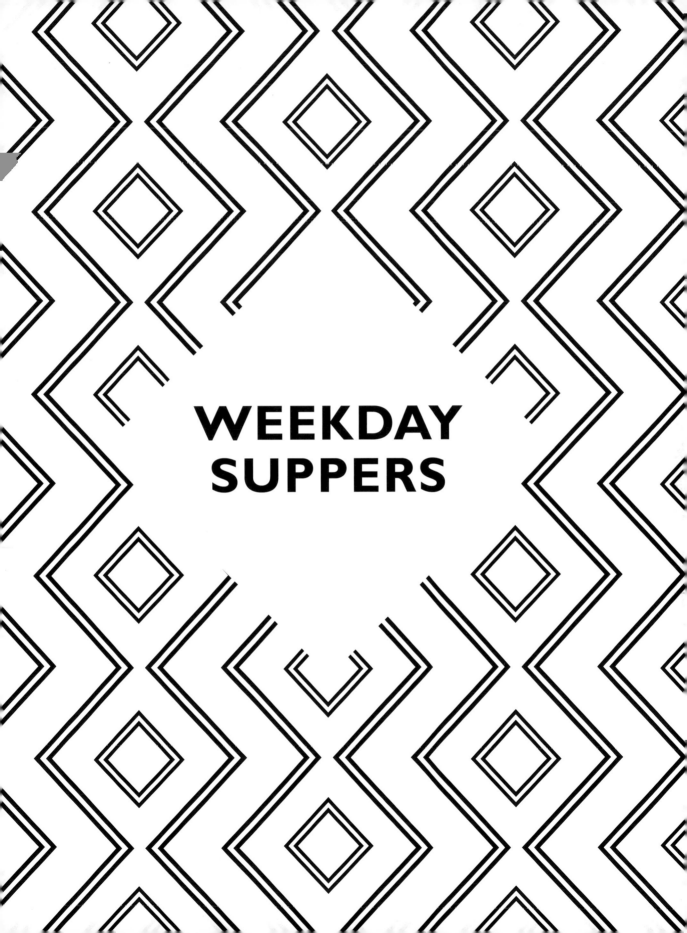

WEEKDAY SUPPERS

Ribollita

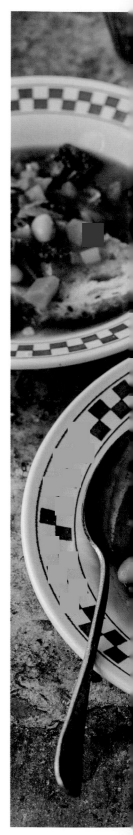

SERVES ⟩⟩⟩ **4–6**

Preparation time ⟩ 15 minutes

Cooking time ⟩ 35 minutes

3 tbsp extra virgin olive oil, plus extra
for drizzling

2 onions, finely chopped

2 celery stalks, diced

2 carrots, diced

1 good-size turnip, peeled and diced

270g/9½oz cavolo nero or kale,
trimmed, stalks sliced and leaves
shredded

½ tsp fennel seeds

½ tsp dried chilli/hot pepper flakes

1 large bay leaf

4 garlic cloves, finely chopped

1 large handful of chopped parsley
leaves and stems

400g/14oz can chopped tomatoes

400g/14oz can cannellini beans, drained

750ml/26fl oz/3¼ cups vegetable stock

4–6 thick slices of slightly stale country-
style bread

sea salt and freshly ground black
pepper

freshly grated Parmesan cheese, to
serve (optional)

This Italian peasant-style soup-cum-stew is a favourite way of utilizing vegetables as well as bread that's marginally stale. Traditionally made in large quantities in advance and then reheated when needed – hence the name ribollita or 're-boiled' – the soup makes a hearty, warming meal. You could also try swapping the bread for pasta to make a minestrone-style soup – either way, it's perfect sustaining comfort food.

⟩⟩⟩ Heat the oil in a large heavy-based saucepan over a medium heat. Add the onions, celery, carrots, turnip and cavolo nero stalks, then turn the heat down slightly and sweat the vegetables for 10 minutes, covered and stirring occasionally, until softened but not browned Stir in the fennel seeds, chilli/hot pepper flakes, bay leaf, garlic and parsley.

⟩⟩⟩ Add the tomatoes, cannellini beans and stock and top up with extra water if the liquid doesn't quite cover the vegetables. Bring to the boil, then turn the heat down and simmer, part-covered, stirring occasionally, for 15 minutes.

⟩⟩⟩ Add the cavolo nero leaves, season with salt and pepper and cook for a further 10 minutes, uncovered, until tender. Add more water if the soup is too thick, but bear in mind that this is a substantial soup.

⟩⟩⟩ Place a slice of bread in the bottom of each serving bowl, ladle the soup over and serve drizzled with extra olive oil. A sprinkling of Parmesan wouldn't go amiss.

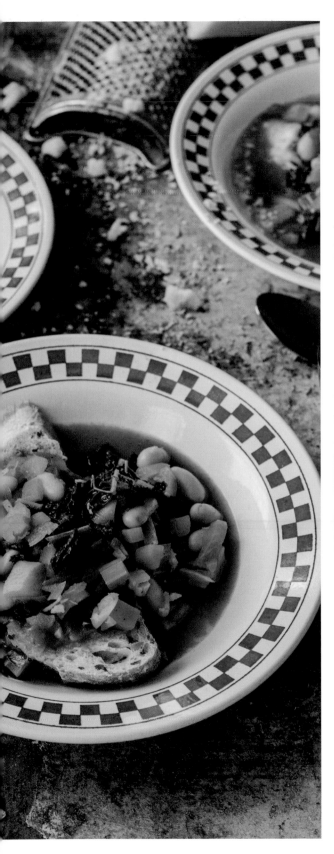

PART-TIME VARIATION
»»» Ribollita with ham hock

A smoked ham hock is economical to buy as well as generous, providing meat as well as creating a decent-flavoured stock. It does need time to cook, so it's perhaps unfeasible to start this soup from scratch on a weekday, so for the sake of convenience add **250g/9oz cooked, shredded ham hock** to the soup with the cavolo nero leaves and continue to cook as described on the previous page.

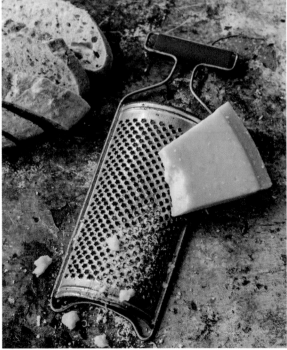

White bean soup WITH cumin carrot mash

SERVES ⟩⟩⟩ **4**

Preparation time ⟩ 15 minutes
Cooking time ⟩ 25 minutes

2 tbsp olive oil
2 onions, finely chopped
2 carrots, thinly sliced
1 celery stalk, thinly sliced
2 bay leaves
1 potato, peeled and cubed
1.2litres/40fl oz/5 cups vegetable stock,
    plus extra if needed
2 x 400g/14oz cans butter beans,
    drained
1 tbsp ground coriander
1 tsp harissa paste
a squeeze of lemon juice
sea salt and freshly ground black
    pepper
humous and warm pitta bread,
    to serve

⟩⟩⟩ **Cumin carrot mash**
1½ tbsp butter
4 carrots, finely chopped
2 garlic cloves, chopped
1 tsp cumin seeds

This is loosely based on *b'sarra*, a Moroccan broad/fava bean soup and popular street food. There are also Egyptian versions of the soup that are made with different types of bean, or with a reduced amount of stock to make a substantial bean dip. To turn this soup into a dip, reduce the amount of stock by two-thirds and blend until smooth and creamy. The cumin carrot mash is my addition and lends texture, flavour and extra substance to the soup.

⟩⟩⟩ Heat half the oil in a large heavy-based saucepan over a medium heat and sauté the onions, carrots and celery for 5 minutes, covered and stirring occasionally, until softened. Add the bay leaves, potato, stock and beans and bring to the boil, then turn the heat down and simmer for 20 minutes, part-covered, until reduced and thickened.

⟩⟩⟩ Stir in the ground coriander, harissa and a squeeze of lemon juice, then season with salt and pepper. Remove the pan from the heat and, using a stick/immersion blender, purée the soup until fairly thick, smooth and creamy, adding more stock if needed.

⟩⟩⟩ Meanwhile, make the cumin carrot mash. Heat the remaining oil with the butter in a saucepan over a medium-low heat. Add the carrots and cook, covered, for 15 minutes until very tender. Add the garlic and cumin and cook for a further 2 minutes, stirring. Season with salt and pepper and mash roughly with the back of a fork. Top the soup with a spoonful of the carrot mash and add a squeeze of lemon juice and a grinding of black pepper. Serve with humous and warm pitta bread on the side.

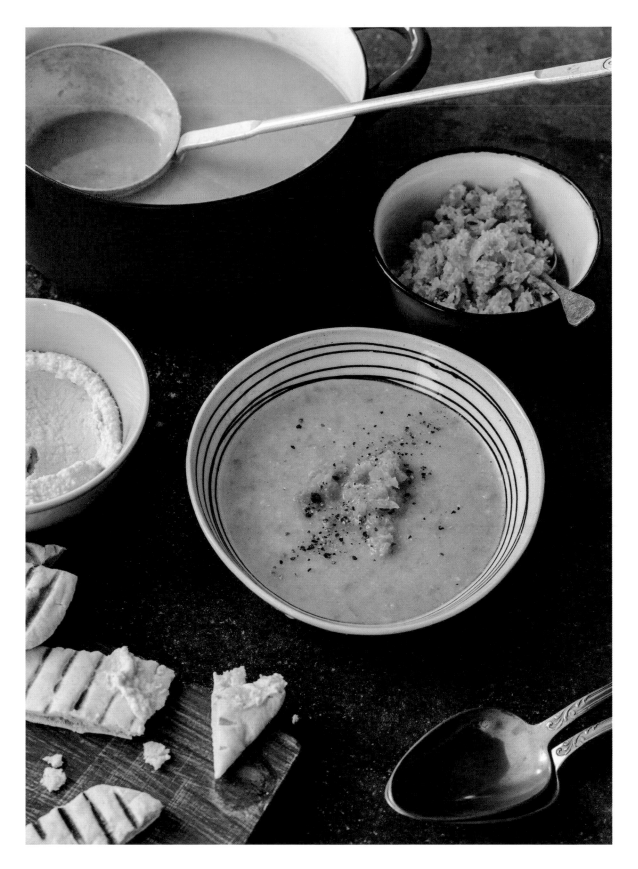

Seaweed AND kamut salad

SERVES ⟩⟩⟩ 4

Preparation time ⟩ 15 minutes

Cooking time ⟩ 15 minutes

100g/3½oz/scant ½ cup kamut or
    barley, short-grain brown rice,
    spelt or freekeh

30g/1oz dried dulse seaweed, rinsed,
    or nori sheets, cut into strips

125g/4½oz long-stem broccoli, stalks
    trimmed

3 tbsp sunflower seeds

1 tsp soy sauce

3 spring onions/scallions, diagonally
    sliced

55g/2oz mixed sprouted beans
    and seeds

10cm/4in piece of cucumber,
    quartered lengthways, deseeded
    and cut into large cubes

1 recipe quantity Japanese-style Tahini
    Dressing (see page 101)

A substantial salad with the feel-good factor. Kamut, also known as Khorasan, is related to an ancient type of wheat and is partnered in this salad with dulse seaweed. Sea vegetables are much under-used, including by me, but their versatility, unique flavour and nutritional value means they have much to offer. Dulse is relatively mild in flavour compared with some other sea vegetables. That said, it takes on a savoury bacon quality when dry fried. Find both kamut and dulse in health food shops and a growing number of large supermarkets.

⟩⟩⟩ Put the kamut in a saucepan and cover with plenty of water. Bring to the boil over a high heat, then turn the heat down and simmer for 15 minutes, part-covered, or until tender. Drain and refresh under cold running water.

⟩⟩⟩ Meanwhile, soak the dulse in just-boiled water for 2 minutes until tender, then drain and roughly chop. Leave to one side. Steam the broccoli for 2 minutes until just tender, then refresh under cold running water. Drain, then slice the stalks, leaving the florets intact.

⟩⟩⟩ Put the sunflower seeds in a large dry frying pan over a medium heat and toast for 2–3 minutes, tossing the pan occasionally. Add the soy sauce and stir until the seeds are coated.

⟩⟩⟩ Put the kamut in a serving dish with the dulse, broccoli, spring onions/scallions, mixed sprouts and cucumber. Spoon the dressing over and toss until everything is combined. Serve sprinkled with the toasted sunflower seeds.

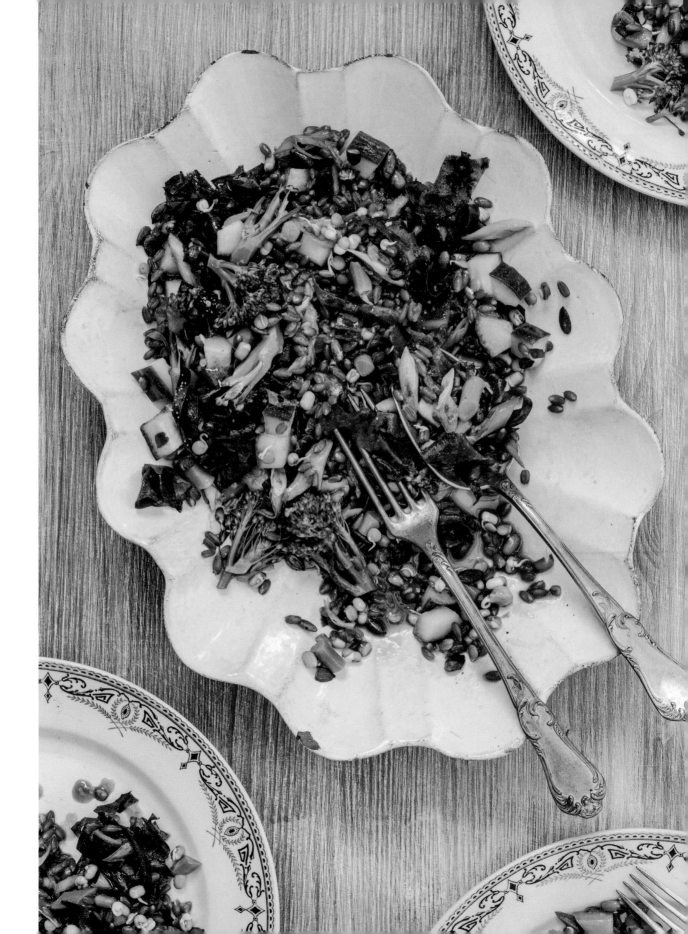

DRESSINGS

A dressing has the ability to bring a salad to life. It not only adds flavour and texture, it can often unify a sometimes disparate selection of ingredients, whether they be fresh vegetables, beans, grains, nuts, pasta or noodles. The best dressings shouldn't mask or dominate a salad but enhance the main ingredients and bring out their flavour.

For me, you can't beat a simple dressing of extra virgin olive oil, lemon juice and a touch of sea salt. It's also the perfect foundation for other additions, such as herbs, spices, citrus zest, mustard and honey. With any dressing, it's best to use the highest-quality ingredients you can afford, so for starters it pays to splash out on a good bottle of extra virgin olive oil and wine vinegar. It's also worth experimenting with different types of oil, including nut and avocado oil, as well as vinegar, including balsamic and sherry.

This small selection of recipes highlights the main types of dressings: oil-based, as in the Caper and Herb Oil and Sesame and Lime Dressing; creamy, such as the Tahini Dressing (two ways) as well as the Feta and Yogurt Dressing; plus oil-free, including the Vietnamese Ginger Chilli Dressing, which is based on rice wine vinegar.

Don't restrict the use of these dressings to just salads. They are also delicious spooned over roasted or steamed vegetables, rice, quinoa, pulses, pasta and noodles.

››› Caper and herb oil

This vibrant dressing is just as good spooned over tomato, bean, grain or leafy green salads as it is over cooked rice or pasta. Mix together 4 tbsp extra virgin olive oil, 3 tbsp capers, drained and roughly chopped, 1 large handful of chopped mixed herbs, such as basil, oregano and thyme, 1 crushed small garlic clove and the juice of ½ lemon.

⟫⟫⟫ Sesame and lime dressing

Mix together 2 tbsp sesame oil, 2 tbsp cold-pressed rapeseed/canola oil and 1cm/½in piece peeled and finely diced fresh root ginger with the finely grated zest of ½ lime and juice of 1½ limes. Season with sea salt and freshly ground black pepper and spoon over Asian-style noodle, grain and vegetable dishes.

⟫⟫⟫ Vietnamese ginger chilli dressing

Perfect over Asian noodle salads, this dressing combines 5 tbsp rice wine vinegar with 4 tsp caster/granulated sugar, ½ tsp ground or finely chopped fresh root ginger and 1 red chilli, deseeded and diced.

⟫⟫⟫ Tahini dressing (two ways)

Tahini is perhaps surprisingly used in Japanese cooking as well as the more familiar European and Middle Eastern dishes. This Japanese-style dressing is good drizzled over griddled/grilled or steamed vegetables as well as noodles or grains. Combine 4 tbsp light soy sauce, 4 tbsp cold-pressed rapeseed/canola oil or similar light oil, 2 tbsp tahini and 4 tsp maple syrup.

For a North African-inspired tahini dressing, mix together 2 tbsp tahini with 2 tbsp plain yogurt, 1 small crushed garlic clove, juice of ½ lemon and ½ tsp clear honey or date syrup.

⟫⟫⟫ Feta and yogurt dressing

Spoon this tangy, creamy dressing over cooked new potatoes, eggs or bean or grain salads. Put 70g/2½oz/heaped ½ cup crumbled feta cheese, 4 tbsp plain yogurt and the juice of ½ lemon in a blender and process until smooth and creamy. Transfer to a bowl and stir in 1 crushed small clove garlic and 4 tbsp finely chopped mint leaves. Season with freshly ground black pepper.

Vietnamese crispy tofu AND cashew salad

SERVES ⟫⟫ **4**

Preparation time ⟫ 20 minutes
Cooking time ⟫ 7 minutes

125g/4½oz rice vermicelli noodles
1 recipe quantity Vietnamese Ginger
    Chilli Dressing (see page 101)
2 carrots, halved crossways and thinly
    sliced into strips
1 small cucumber, quartered
    lengthways, deseeded, and thinly
    sliced into strips
2 handfuls of shredded red cabbage
1 red pepper, deseeded and thinly
    sliced
3 spring onions/scallions, thinly sliced
2 handfuls of chopped mint leaves
2 handfuls of torn basil leaves
250g/9oz crisp fried tofu pieces, halved
    if large
1 Little Gem/Bibb lettuce, leaves
    separated
70g/2½oz/heaped ½ cup salted
    roasted cashew nuts

Sweet, sour, hot, spicy and salty, this vibrant salad includes all five elements that are fundamental to Vietnamese cooking. Vital, too, is the contrast in textures, from the crunch of the cashews to the crisp vegetables and soft, yielding rice noodles. Find crisp fried tofu in Asian grocers or cook your own following the instructions below. Alternatively, try the soy-glazed chicken option, opposite, if you are serving to non-vegetarians.

⟫⟫ Put the noodles in a large mixing bowl, cover with just-boiled water from a kettle and stir, then cover with a plate and leave to stand for 3 minutes, or until tender. Drain and refresh under cold running water, drain again and put in a large serving bowl. Spoon the dressing over and toss until thoroughly combined.

⟫⟫ Add the carrots, cucumber, cabbage, pepper, spring onions/scallions and half the herbs to the bowl containing the noodles and toss until combined.

⟫⟫ Heat a large dry, non-stick frying pan over a medium heat and cook the tofu for 2–4 minutes, turning regularly, until warmed through and crisped up. (If you can't find crisp fried tofu, fry 250g/9oz cubed tofu in 3 tablespoons sunflower oil, turning occasionally, until golden and crisp. Drain on paper towels.)

⟫⟫ Arrange the lettuce leaves on a large serving plate and top with the noodle salad, remaining herbs, cashews and crisp tofu before serving.

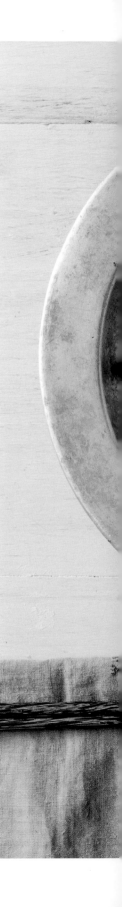

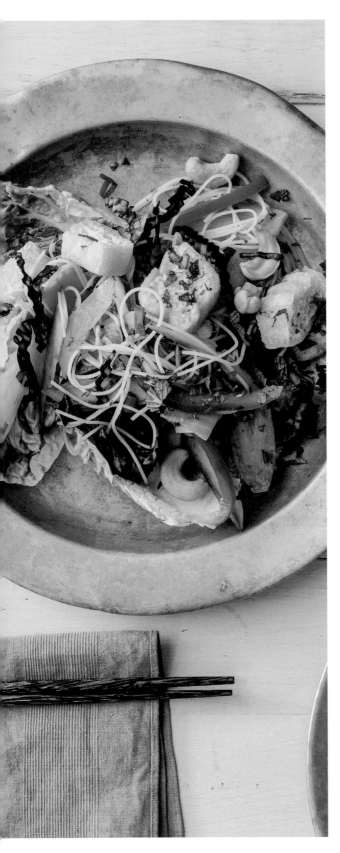

PART-TIME VARIATION

››› Chicken and peanut Vietnamese salad

This is a perfect way to use up cooked leftover roast meat or, if you are starting from scratch, cut **400g/14oz skinless, boneless chicken breasts** or **pork fillet** into thin strips. Fry in **1 tbsp sunflower oil** for 5 minutes, or until cooked through. Add **1 tbsp light soy sauce** and cook briefly until golden. When making the dressing, replace 1 tbsp rice vinegar with **1 tbsp fish sauce**. Serve sprinkled with **70g/2½oz/¾ cup chopped salted peanuts** in place of the cashews.

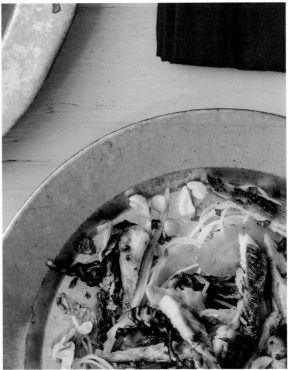

Roasted vegetables WITH skorthalia

SERVES ››› **4**

Preparation time › 15 minutes

Cooking time › 40 minutes

5 tbsp extra virgin olive oil

2 tbsp balsamic vinegar

2 red onions, halved and each half cut
    into 3 wedges

1 red pepper, halved, deseeded and cut
    into long wedges

1 orange pepper, halved, deseeded and
    cut into long wedges

8 baby courgettes/zucchini, halved
    lengthways

100g/3½oz drained bottled artichokes

sea salt and freshly ground black
    pepper

150g/5½oz crumbled feta cheese and
    1 handful of Greek basil leaves,
    to serve

››› Skorthalia

6 garlic cloves, unpeeled

4 slices of day-old white bread, crusts
    removed, torn into pieces

70g/2½oz/⅓ cup blanched almonds

juice of 1 small lemon

milk, if needed

Skorthalia is a rich and creamy Greek sauce-cum-dip made with bread, almonds, lemon juice and more than a hint of garlic. You can use raw garlic, but to make the most of the oven while cooking the vegetables, the garlic is roasted here for a more subtly flavoured sauce. Greek basil has smaller leaves than the regular variety and a slightly stronger flavour, but you can choose whatever is to hand, or indeed use fresh thyme, oregano or marjoram.

››› Mix together 2 tablespoons of the olive oil with the balsamic vinegar in a large bowl. Season and add the onions, peppers and courgettes/zucchini, then turn to coat them in the marinade. Leave to marinate while the oven is heating up.

››› Preheat the oven to 200°C/400°F/Gas 6. Tip the marinated vegetables into two large roasting pans, spreading them out into an even layer, and add the garlic cloves for the skorthalia. Roast for 20 minutes, or until the garlic is soft – give it a little squeeze. Remove the garlic, turn the vegetables and add the artichokes. Return to the oven for a further 15–20 minutes, or until the vegetables are tender and blackened in places.

››› Meanwhile, to make the skorthalia, soak the bread in 300ml/10½fl oz/scant 1¼ cups water. Grind the almonds in a food processor. Squeeze the roasted garlic out of its papery skin and add to processor with the soaked bread and lemon juice. Blend to a smooth, creamy consistency, then gradually pour in the remaining olive oil until thickened to the consistency of mayonnaise. If the sauce is too thick, add a little milk to loosen it, then season generously with salt and pepper.

››› Spoon the skorthalia onto plates and serve with the roasted vegetables, feta and sprinkled with basil.

PART-TIME VARIATION
››› Smoked mackerel with skorthalia

Fillets of **smoked mackerel** are economical to buy and require little effort – perfect for a weekday meal. Try flavouring the mackerel with a spice mix, such as **harissa**, then cook in a frying pan – no need to add extra oil – until the skin is crisp and the fish is warmed through. Add a **squeeze of lemon juice** and serve with the skorthalia, as described above.

Roasted mushrooms ON white bean mash

Harissa paste, a vibrant North African blend of chilli and spices, makes a quick and easy marinade for the portabellini mushrooms as well as the lamb steak variation, while the salsa topping adds crunch and colour to both options. You could also try a spoonful of Romesco Sauce (see page 201) or the North African-inspired Tahini Dressing (see page 101) instead of the salsa with the mushrooms or indeed the lamb.

››› Preheat the oven to 190°C/375°F/Gas 5. To make the white bean mash, wrap the whole garlic bulb in foil and roast in the oven for 25 minutes, or until the cloves are tender.

››› Meanwhile, mix together half the olive oil with the harissa paste and season with salt and pepper. Brush the mixture over the caps of the mushrooms. Put the mushrooms in a large roasting pan, gill-side up, and roast for 20 minutes, or until tender.

››› While the garlic and mushrooms are roasting, continue with the white bean mash. Put the butter beans in a pan with the remaining olive oil, lemon juice, ground coriander and 3 tablespoons water and cook over a gentle heat for 5 minutes until softened. When ready, squeeze the roast garlic out of its papery skin into the pan and mash everything to a rough purée. Season well with salt and pepper.

››› Spoon the mash onto plates and top with the mushrooms and any juices in the pan. Serve topped with the salsa and a rocket/arugula salad by the side.

PART-TIME VARIATION
››› Lamb with white bean mash

Instead of the mushrooms, brush **4 lamb leg steaks** with the olive oil and harissa mixture. Season with salt and pepper and leave to marinate for about 30 minutes. Heat a large griddle/grill pan over a high heat and griddle the lamb for 2–3 minutes on each side, or until cooked to your liking. Remove the lamb from the griddle/grill pan, cover with foil and leave to rest for 5 minutes before serving on top of the white bean mash. Serve topped with the salsa and a rocket/arugula salad by the side.

SERVES ››› **4**
Preparation time ᴐ 20 minutes
Cooking time ᴐ 25 minutes

4 tbsp extra virgin olive oil
1 tbsp harissa paste
350g/12oz portabellini mushrooms
1 recipe quantity Jalapeño Tomato
    Salsa (see page 66)
rocket/arugula salad, to serve
sea salt and freshly ground black
    pepper

››› **White bean mash**
1 large garlic bulb, top trimmed
    horizontally
2 x 400g/14oz cans butter beans,
    drained
juice of 1 lemon
2 tsp ground coriander

Smoky aubergines
<u>WITH</u> polenta

SERVES ⟩⟩⟩ **4**

Preparation time ⟩ 20 minutes
Cooking time ⟩ 30 minutes

4 tbsp extra virgin olive oil
4 tsp balsamic vinegar
6–8 baby aubergines/eggplants,
    depending on size, halved
    lengthways, leaving the stem
    attached, or 2 aubergines/
    eggplants, cubed
200g/7oz/1⅓ cups instant polenta/
    cornmeal
1½ tbsp butter
25g/1oz/⅓ cup finely grated Parmesan
    cheese
1 handful of flaked/slivered almonds,
    toasted (see method on page 22)
sea salt and freshly ground black
    pepper

⟩⟩⟩ **Chipotle dressing**

1 dried chipotle chilli
1 garlic clove, finely chopped
½ red onion, finely chopped
40g/1½oz chopped coriander/cilantro
    leaves
juice of ½ lime
1 tsp caster/granulated sugar

Aubergines/eggplants work so well with the comforting texture of the soft, creamy polenta/cornmeal. Chipotle chillies, or dried jalapeños, give a lovely smoky heat to this dish – simply soak them in a small amount of just-boiled water until softened. You could use 2–3 teaspoons chipotle paste or 1 teaspoon smoked hot paprika instead, if you prefer.

⟩⟩⟩ To make the dressing, soak the chipotle chilli in 4 tablespoons just-boiled water and leave to steep for 20 minutes until softened.

⟩⟩⟩ Meanwhile, turn the grill/broiler to high. Mix together 3 tablespoons of the olive oil with the balsamic vinegar in a roasting dish. Season with salt and pepper, add the aubergines/eggplants and turn until coated in the marinade. Grill/broil for 20–30 minutes, turning once or twice, until tender and blackened in places.

⟩⟩⟩ To finish the dressing, drain the chipotle, reserving the soaking water, and roughly chop. Discard the seeds and put the chipotle in a pestle and mortar, then grind to a paste with the garlic and a large pinch of sea salt. Transfer to a bowl and stir in the onion and coriander/cilantro. Mix together the lime juice, sugar and the remaining oil and stir the mixture into the chipotle. Leave to one side.

⟩⟩⟩ To make the polenta/cornmeal, bring 850ml/29fl oz/scant 3½ cups water and the chipotle soaking water to the boil in a saucepan. Gradually pour in the polenta/cornmeal, stirring constantly with a wooden spoon, and cook for 8 minutes, or until it has thickened to the consistency of mashed potato. Stir in the butter and Parmesan and season with salt and pepper. Spoon the polenta/cornmeal onto serving plates and top with the aubergine/eggplant and the chipotle dressing. Scatter the almonds over the dish before serving.

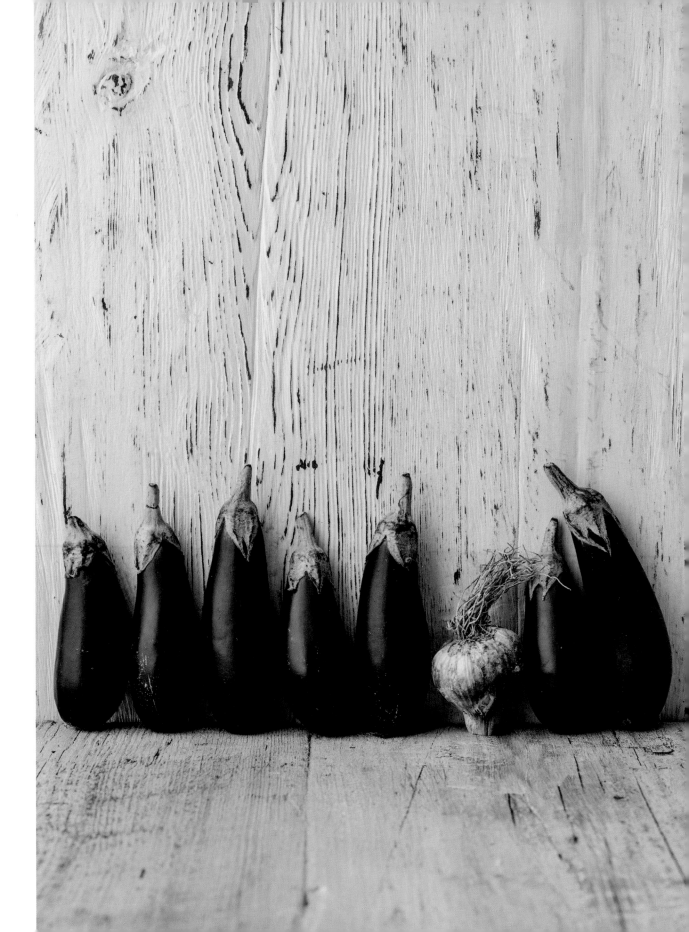

Lemon roast vegetables
WITH scamorza

SERVES »»» 4

Preparation time » 20 minutes

Cooking time » 40 minutes

2 tbsp extra virgin olive oil

finely grated zest and juice of
    1 large lemon

1 tsp turmeric

1 tsp dried chilli/hot pepper flakes

800g/1lb 12oz white potatoes, such
    as Maris Piper, cut into bite-size
    chunks (no need to peel)

2 onions, halved and cut into wedges

250g/9oz cherry tomatoes

1 fennel bulb, quartered lengthways,
    fronds reserved

200g/7oz scamorza or mozzarella
    cheese, cut into chunks

4 tbsp pumpkin seeds, toasted
    (see method on page 71)

1 recipe quantity Caper and Herb Oil
    (see page 100)

sea salt and freshly ground black
    pepper

This is my kind of recipe – pretty much everything is mixed together and then just put in the oven and left to cook. Scamorza can best be described as a type of smoked mozzarella, but it is interchangeable with regular mozzarella or any other type of 'melting' cheese. There is also the white fish variation, below, which can be cooked in the oven at the same time as the potatoes. The summery flavoured oil adds a vibrant lift to both the vegetarian and fish dishes.

»»» Preheat the oven to 220°C/425°F/Gas 7. Mix together the olive oil, the lemon zest and juice, the turmeric and chilli/hot pepper flakes in a large mixing bowl. Add the potatoes and turn until coated in the lemony spice mix. Divide the potatoes and any marinade between two large roasting pans, cover with foil and roast for 20 minutes.

»»» Add the onions, tomatoes and fennel to the roasting pans, season with salt and pepper and turn until combined. Return to the oven and cook, uncovered, for a further 20 minutes, or until the potatoes are starting to crisp and the vegetables are tender.

»»» Top the roasted potatoes and vegetables with the scamorza, pumpkin seeds and fennel fronds, then drizzle the caper and herb oil over before serving.

PART-TIME VARIATION
»»» White fish with caper and herb oil

Lightly oil 4 sheets of baking paper, each large enough to make a parcel. Place **4 thick fillets white fish, such as pollock**, on top of the paper, season with salt and pepper, add a **squeeze of lemon juice** and a **few fennel fronds**. Gather up the sides of the paper and fold over at the top to make 4 sealed parcels.

Place the parcels on a baking sheet and roast on the bottom shelf of the oven, below the potatoes and vegetables, for 16–20 minutes, depending on the thickness of the fillets, until the fish flakes easily. Serve on top of the potato mixture in place of the scamorza and pumpkin seeds, with the fennel fronds and the caper and herb oil drizzled over the top.

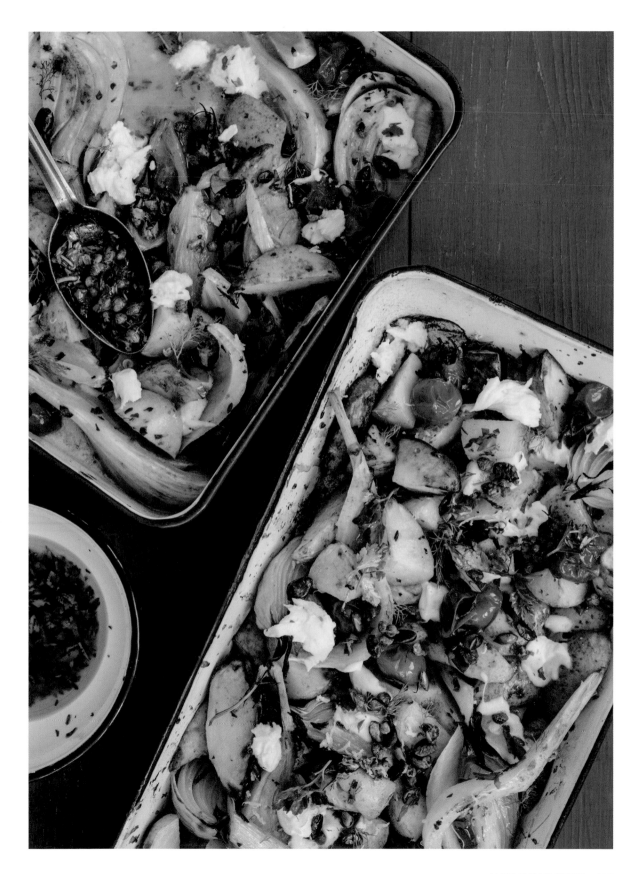

Pan haggerty WITH savoury custard

SERVES ⟫⟫ 4

Preparation time ⟫ 20 minutes

Cooking time ⟫ 40 minutes

2 tbsp butter

2 tbsp olive oil

4 leeks, thinly sliced

100g/3½oz kale, tough stalks
discarded, leaves shredded

650g/1lb 7oz white potatoes, such
as Maris Piper, peeled and thinly
sliced into rounds

1 tsp turmeric

500ml/17fl oz/generous 2 cups
vegetable stock

sea salt and freshly ground black
pepper

⟫⟫ Savoury custard

1 tbsp cornflour/cornstarch

300ml/10½fl oz/1¼ cups milk

2 egg yolks

1 tsp English mustard

150g/5½oz/1½ cups grated mature/
sharp Cheddar cheese

This twist on the traditional British layered potato dish makes a comforting meal for a cold wintery evening. The layers of potato are interspersed with a mixture of leeks and kale and it comes with a savoury cheese custard made with mature Cheddar, although a classic blue cheese, such as Stilton, would also be delicious.

⟫⟫ Heat half the butter and the olive oil in a large non-stick, ovenproof sauté pan and fry the leeks and kale for 5 minutes until tender, then remove from the pan. Arrange half the potatoes in the pan, overlapping them slightly to make an even layer. Spoon the leek and kale mixture on top. Arrange the remaining potatoes on top, again overlapping them to make an even layer.

⟫⟫ Stir the turmeric into the stock, then pour it over the potatoes and season with salt and pepper. Place a round of baking paper on top of the potatoes to stop them drying out and cover the pan with a lid. Bring the stock to the boil, then turn the heat to low and simmer for 20 minutes until the potatoes have softened.

⟫⟫ Meanwhile, make the savoury custard. Mix the cornflour/cornstarch into a little of the milk in a mixing bowl and whisk in the egg yolks. Heat the remaining milk until warm and gradually pour it into the egg yolk mixture, whisking continuously. Return the mixture to the pan and simmer for 6–8 minutes, stirring regularly, until thickened to the consistency of runny custard. Add the mustard and cheese and stir until combined.

⟫⟫ Preheat the grill/broiler to high. Remove the lid and round of paper from the pan containing the potatoes and cook for a further 5–10 minutes until the stock has reduced and the potatoes are tender. Dot the remaining butter over the top and grill/broil for 3–4 minutes until the potatoes turn golden and start to crisp. Serve the potatoes with the savoury custard by the side.

PART-TIME VARIATION

⟫⟫ Pan haggerty with smoked bacon

Put **200g/7oz smoked lardons** or **diced bacon** into a large dry sauté pan and cook over a medium-low heat until the fat starts to run, then turn the heat to medium and fry for another 5 minutes until golden and crisp. Remove from the pan with a slotted spoon, drain on kitchen paper and scatter over the top of the pan haggerty before serving.

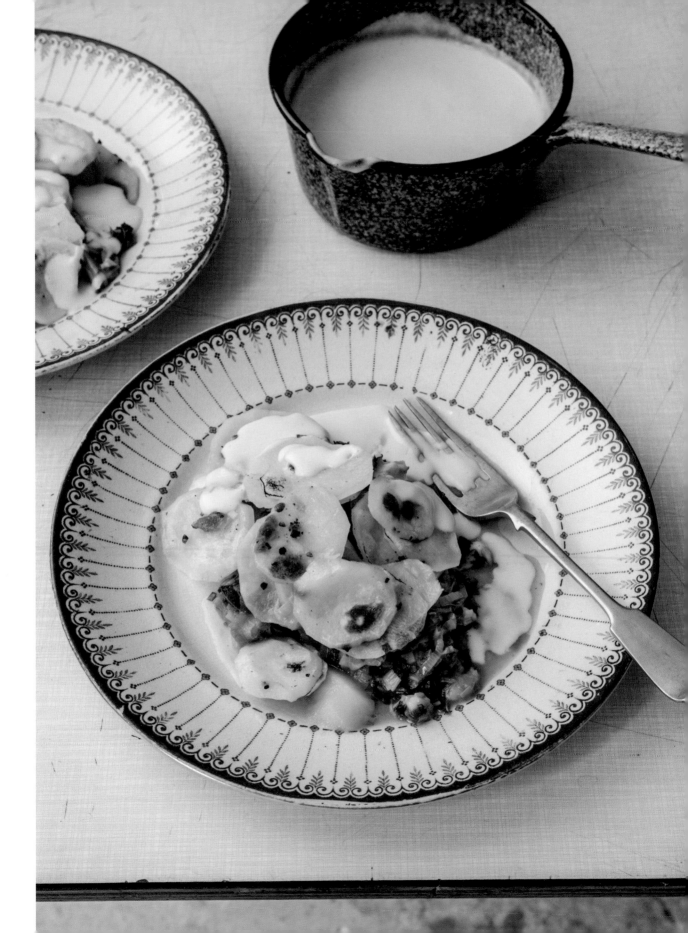

Pan-fried gnocchi
<u>WITH</u> chimichurri sauce

SERVES ⟫⟫ **4**

Preparation time ⟫ 20 minutes

Cooking time ⟫ 10 minutes

2 handfuls of blanched hazelnuts

2 tbsp olive oil

800g/1lb 12oz fresh ready-made
   gnocchi

4 vine-ripened tomatoes, deseeded
   and diced

2 large handfuls of pea shoots,
   to serve

⟫⟫⟫ **Chimichurri sauce**

1 large bunch of flat-leaf parsley leaves,
   finely chopped

1 large bunch of oregano leaves, finely
   chopped

2 garlic cloves, crushed

1 red chilli, deseeded and finely
   chopped

juice of ½ lemon

4 tbsp extra virgin olive oil

1 tbsp white wine vinegar

½ tsp sea salt

Fragrant and fiery, chimichurri is the Argentinian equivalent of Italian pesto and makes a lively sauce, marinade or dip for all types of dishes. For a speedy light meal, the sauce is served spooned over parcels of crisp fried gnocchi. You could also add a can of chickpeas and warm through with the gnocchi for extra substance, or serve with steak instead of the hazelnuts.

⟫⟫⟫ To make the chimichurri, put the parsley, oregano, garlic, chilli, lemon juice, olive oil, vinegar and salt in a bowl and stir until combined, then taste and adjust the seasoning, if needed. (The mixture can also be blended in a food processor until finely chopped.) Leave to one side for about 10 minutes to allow the flavours to mingle.

⟫⟫⟫ Meanwhile, put the hazelnuts in a large dry, non-stick frying pan over a medium heat and toast for 5 minutes, tossing occasionally, until starting to colour. Remove from the pan, then roughly chop and leave to cool.

⟫⟫⟫ Heat the olive oil in the frying pan over a medium heat and fry the gnocchi for 2–3 minutes until golden and starting to crisp (you may need to do this in two batches).

⟫⟫⟫ Stir the tomatoes into the pan and warm through for a minute, then add enough of the chimichurri to coat the gnocchi. (Store any leftover chimichurri in an airtight container in the refrigerator for up to 1 week.) To serve, scatter the hazelnuts over the gnocchi and top with the pea shoots.

PART-TIME VARIATION
⟫⟫⟫ Steak and chimichurri gnocchi

Brush **2 fillet or sirloin steaks, about 250g/9oz each**, with seasoned olive oil. Heat a griddle/grill or large, heavy-based frying pan over a high heat and sear the steaks for 2–3 minutes on each side, turning once or twice. Cover and leave to rest for 5 minutes before cutting into slices and serving in place of the hazelnuts.

Paneer, egg <u>AND</u> potato gratin

This potato gratin comes with an Indian twist thanks to the addition of spices and the Asian cheese, paneer. With its slightly dense, crumbly texture and mild flavour, paneer takes to spicing with ease. This makes a satisfyingly simple meal served with a good chunk of crusty bread and perhaps a crisp green side salad.

>>> Preheat the oven to 200°C/400°F/Gas 6. Cook the potatoes in plenty of salted boiling water with half the turmeric for 10–12 minutes until almost tender. Drain the potatoes and leave until cool enough to handle.

>>> Meanwhile, heat 2 tablespoons of the oil in a large non-stick sauté pan over a medium heat and fry the onions for 8 minutes, stirring regularly, until softened. Add the garlic, fennel seeds, cumin seeds, green peppers and chilli and cook for 5 minutes until softened.

>>> Slice the potatoes into 1cm/½in thick slices and add to the pan, turn gently until combined. Add the remaining turmeric to the stock and pour it over the vegetavles in the pan. Bring to the boil over a high heat, then turn the heat down and simmer for 5 minutes until the stock has reduced by three-quarters. Stir in half the coriander/cilantro and transfer to a medium baking dish.

>>> Make four indentations in the potato mixture and break an egg into each one. Scatter the paneer over the top and drizzle with the remaining oil. Season with pepper, cover with foil, then bake for 15 minutes. Remove the foil and cook for a further 5–8 minutes until the egg whites have set but the yolks remain runny. Scatter over the remaining coriander/cilantro and serve with steamed green vegetables.

SERVES >>> 4
Preparation time ∂ 15 minutes
Cooking time ∂ 40 minutes

800g/1lb 12 oz waxy potatoes, such as Charlotte, halved if large (no need to peel)
2 tsp turmeric
3 tbsp coconut or olive oil
2 onions, thinly sliced
2 large garlic cloves, finely chopped
2 tsp fennel seeds
1 tsp cumin seeds
2 large green peppers, deseeded and each cut into 8 strips
1 long green chilli, deseeded and thinly sliced
325ml/11fl oz/generous 1⅓ cups vegetable stock
2 large handfuls of chopped coriander/cilantro leaves
4 large eggs
150g/5½oz/1¼ cups cubed paneer cheese
sea salt and freshly ground black pepper
steamed green vegetables, to serve

Okonomiyaki

SERVES ⟩⟩⟩ **2–4**

Preparation time ⟩ 15 minutes

Cooking time ⟩ 12 minutes

150g/5½oz white cabbage, finely
shredded

6 spring onions/scallions, thinly sliced

50g/1¾oz kohlrabi or turnip, peeled
and coarsely grated

110g/3¾oz/scant 1 cup plain/
all-purpose flour

½ tsp sea salt

2 large eggs, lightly beaten

1½ tbsp sunflower oil

⟩⟩⟩ **Topping**

mayonnaise in a squeezy bottle,
for drizzling

1 handful of radishes, sliced

1 handful of wild garlic leaves (and
flowers) or chives, chopped

1 tbsp pink pickled ginger
(or see recipe page 165)

1 tsp nori flakes

Sometimes referred to as 'Japanese pizza', the name okonomiyaki actually means 'grilled/broiled as you like it', which goes to explain the many regional styles as well as personal variations there are of this dish. Just to confuse matters, okonomiyaki is probably more accurately described as a cross between a thick omelette and a pancake. This interpretation is based on the Osaka-style, where all the ingredients are mixed together before cooking. Try the veggie version, or add meat or fish for non-veggie guests or family.

⟩⟩⟩ Put the cabbage, spring onions/scallions and kohlrabi in a large mixing bowl. Add the flour and salt and stir well until thoroughly combined.

⟩⟩⟩ Mix the eggs with 100ml/3½fl oz/scant ½ cup water. Pour it into the bowl containing the dry ingredients and stir gently but thoroughly until combined. Try to keep the stirring brief as you don't want to activate the gluten in the flour as this will produce a heavy pancake.

⟩⟩⟩ Heat half the oil in a medium non-stick frying pan over a medium heat and tilt the pan so it coats the base. Tip the contents of the bowl into the pan and flatten with a spatula into a thick, round pancake shape, as even as you can get it. Turn the heat down slightly as you don't want the base to burn and cook for 5–6 minutes until light golden.

⟩⟩⟩ Turn the pancake over (the easiest way to do this is to place a large plate on top of the pan and carefully turn it over to release the pancake). At this point, add the remaining oil to the pan before sliding the okonomiyaki back into the pan. Press down with a spatula and cook for another 5–6 minutes until light golden.

⟩⟩⟩ Slide the okonomiyaki onto a chopping board. Drizzle the mayonnaise in lines over the top and pile the radishes, wild garlic, pickled ginger and nori in the middle. Serve cut into wedges.

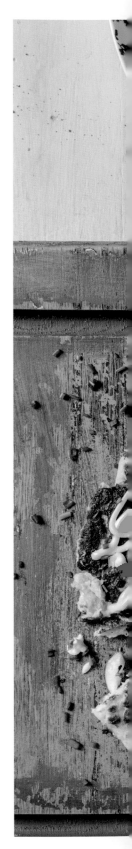

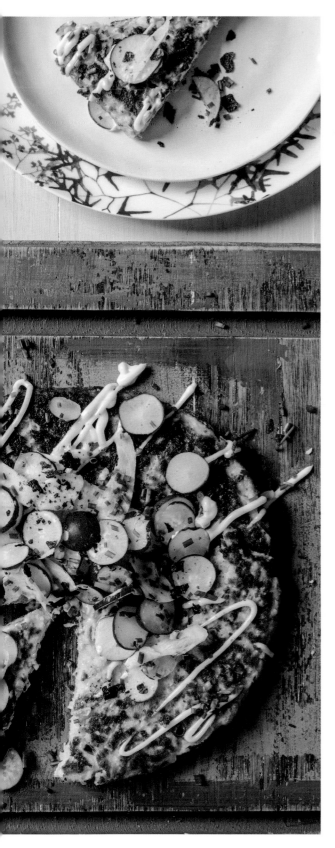

PART-TIME VARIATIONS

There are so many variations on toppings and fillings, so feel free to pick your own or try these suggestions:

⟩⟩⟩ Bonito okonomiyaki

Bonito flakes (paper-thin slices of dried fish similar to tuna) are typical. Sprinkle **2 tbsp bonito flakes** over the top instead of the radishes.

⟩⟩⟩ Bacon okonomiyaki

Put **200/7oz diced bacon** in the dry frying pan and place over a medium-low heat. When the fat starts to run, turn the heat to medium and fry the lardons for 5 minutes until golden and crisp. Stir half into the batter mixture and scatter the remainder over the top. There is no need to clean the pan before adding the okonomiyaki mixture, although you may like to reduce the amount of oil to 1 tablespoon.

⟩⟩⟩ Smoked salmon okonomiyaki

Stir **100g/3½oz smoked salmon pieces** into the batter mixture and top with Japanese pickles.

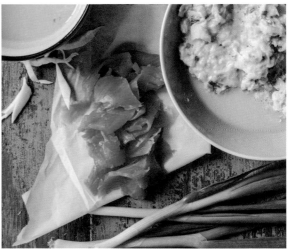

Salt AND Szechuan pepper tofu

SERVES ⟩⟩⟩ **4**

Preparation time ⟩ 15 minutes
Cooking time ⟩ 15 minutes

500g/1lb 2oz block of tofu, drained
    well on paper towels, cut in half
    lengthways and then cut into
    1cm/½in thick slices
1 tsp whole black peppercorns
1 tsp Szechuan pepper
1½ tsp sea salt
125g/4½oz/1¼ cups cornflour/
    cornstarch
2 eggs
sunflower oil, for deep frying
3 spring onions/scallions,
    diagonally sliced
1 red chilli, deseeded and finely sliced
1 lime, cut into wedges
jasmine rice and pak choi/bok choy
    dressed in soy sauce, to serve

Szechuan pepper has a distinctive lemony, peppery heat that spices up the light, crisp battered slices of tofu. It is also a classic with crisp slices of squid. If making both, deep-fry the tofu first. Serve simply with steamed jasmine rice and pak choi/bok choy.

⟩⟩⟩ Arrange the sliced tofu between two layers of paper towels to drain and remove any excess water.

⟩⟩⟩ Meanwhile, put the black peppercorns and Szechuan pepper in a large non-stick frying pan over a medium heat and toast for 1–2 minutes, tossing the pan frequently, until they smell aromatic. Grind the spices and salt to a powder in a pestle and mortar or mini food processor.

⟩⟩⟩ Put the cornflour/cornstarch into a shallow bowl and stir in the ground spice mixture. Lightly beat the eggs in a second shallow bowl.

⟩⟩⟩ Heat enough oil to half-fill a wok or pan over a medium heat (it's hot enough when a cube of bread turns golden in 35 seconds). Dip each slice of tofu into the egg and then the cornflour/cornstarch mixture until coated all over. Fry in batches, turning once, for 3 minutes until golden and crisp all over. Drain on paper towels and keep warm in a low oven while you prepare all of the tofu.

⟩⟩⟩ Scatter the spring onions/scallions and chilli over the tofu and serve with wedges of lime, jasmine rice and pak choi/bok choy by the side.

PART-TIME VARIATION
⟩⟩⟩ Salt and Szechuan pepper squid

Rinse **500g/1lb 2oz prepared squid** (about 12 small squid). Cut off the tentacles, if attached, and open out the body of each squid. Prepare the squid and tentacles as for the tofu, above, and cook for 30 seconds until the batter is crisp and golden, then drain on paper towels. Serve as suggested above.

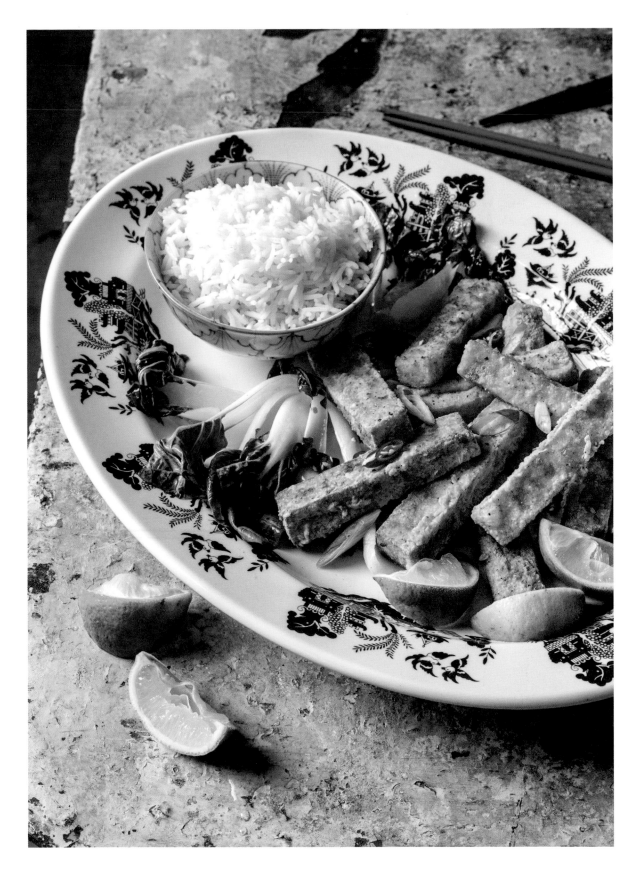

Noodle pot <u>WITH</u> Thai pesto

SERVES ⟫⟫ **4**
Preparation time ⟩ 20 minutes
Cooking time ⟩ 15 minutes

700ml/24fl oz/3 cups vegetable stock
300ml/10½fl oz/1¼ cups coconut milk
1 large sweet potato, peeled and cut
    into bite-size pieces
2 long lemongrass stalks, outer leaves
    removed and inside bruised
4 kaffir lime leaves
4cm/1½in piece of fresh root
    ginger, peeled and thickly sliced
185g/6½oz wholewheat noodles
165g/5¾oz chestnut/cremini
    mushrooms, thinly sliced
5 large handfuls of baby spinach leaves

⟫⟫ Thai pesto
50g/1¾oz/scant ½ cup cashew nuts,
    finely chopped
1 large bunch of Thai basil leaves or
    regular basil, torn into pieces
1 garlic clove, chopped
1cm/½in piece of fresh root ginger,
    peeled and finely grated
juice of ½ lime
3 tbsp cold-pressed rapeseed/
    canola oil
1 red chilli, deseeded and finely
    chopped
sea salt and freshly ground black
    pepper

Don't let the long list of ingredients put you off as this comforting coconut noodle broth couldn't be easier to make. The Thai pesto adds the finishing touch and any left over will keep in an airtight jar in the refrigerator for up to a week – just cover the top with extra oil.

⟫⟫ To make the Thai pesto, grind the cashews, basil, garlic and ginger in a pestle and mortar or mini food processor to a coarse paste. Pour in the lime juice and oil, season and continue to grind until almost smooth. Stir in the chilli and 1 tablespoon water to loosen the pesto slightly, then leave to one side.

⟫⟫ Pour the stock and coconut milk into a large saucepan and add the sweet potato, lemongrass, lime leaves and ginger. Bring to the boil, then turn the heat down and simmer for 10 minutes, part-covered and stirring occasionally, until the sweet potato is almost tender.

⟫⟫ Meanwhile, cook the noodles following the instructions on the pack, drain and refresh under cold running water. Leave to one side.

⟫⟫ Add the mushrooms and spinach to the coconut broth, stir until combined and cook over a medium-low heat for 5 minutes until the vegetables are tender. Pick out the lemongrass, ginger and lime leaves, stir in the noodles and warm through. Season with salt and pepper and serve in large shallow bowls topped with a good spoonful of the pesto. (Spoon any leftover pesto into a jar and keep in the refrigerator for up to 1 week.)

PART-TIME VARIATION
⟫⟫ Prawn/shrimp and red pepper noodle pot

For a speedy seafood alternative, swap the mushrooms and sweet potato for prawns/shrimp and red pepper. Add **1 large deseeded and sliced red pepper**, **625ml/21½fl oz/2⅔ cups stock** and **6 handfuls of spinach** along with the lemongrass, lime leaves and ginger to the pan with the coconut milk, **2 tsp fish sauce** and ½ tsp caster/granulated sugar. Simmer for 10 minutes until the pepper is tender. Add **300g/10½oz raw king prawns/jumbo shrimp** and the cooked noodles and cook for another 3 minutes until the prawns/shrimps are pink and cooked through. Serve topped with the Thai pesto.

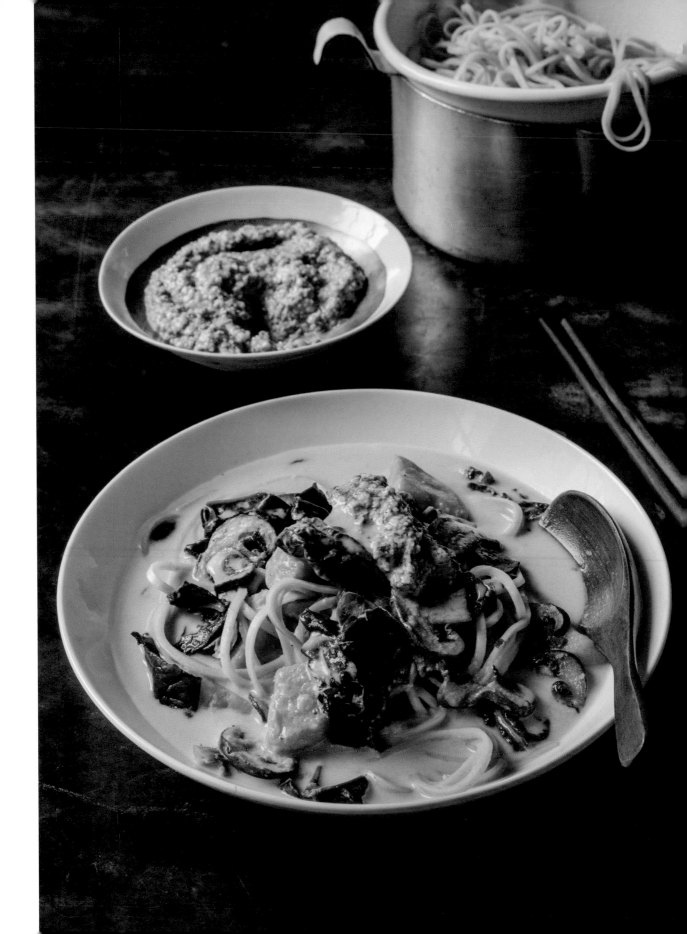

Baked avocado
<u>WITH</u> chilli beans

SERVES ⟫⟫⟫ 4

Preparation time ⟩ 15 minutes
Cooking time ⟩ 18 minutes

2 large avocados, halved and pitted
juice of ½ lime
4 eggs
sea salt and freshly ground black
    pepper
4 corn flatbreads, warmed, to serve

⟫⟫⟫ **Chilli beans**

2 tbsp olive oil, plus extra for drizzling
5 spring onions/scallions, sliced
1 red pepper, deseeded
2 garlic cloves, finely chopped
400g/14oz can kidney beans, drained
    and rinsed
4 good-size, vine-ripened tomatoes,
    quartered, deseeded and chopped
½ tsp dried chilli/hot pepper flakes
2 tsp ground coriander
1 tsp ground cumin
2 handfuls of roughly chopped
    coriander/cilantro leaves
juice of ½ lime

This makes a satisfying and nutritious midweek meal served with warm flatbreads. A halved, pitted avocado makes the perfect container for an egg, which is baked until the avocado softens and the egg yolk sets slightly. The addition of the chilli beans turns it into a filling meal.

⟫⟫⟫ Preheat the oven to 180°C/350°F/Gas 4. Using a teaspoon, scoop out a little flesh from the centre of each avocado (and eat) so you can fit in more of the egg. Squeeze over the lime juice to prevent the avocado browning.

⟫⟫⟫ Break one of the eggs into a bowl and, using a teaspoon, scoop out the yolk and place it in the hole of the avocado, then spoon in the white (you may not be able to use it all and any leftover can be frozen for future use). Season and drizzle over a little oil. Repeat with the remaining avocado halves, lime juice and oil.

⟫⟫⟫ Place the avocado halves in a small baking pan, so they fit snugly (you could use scrunched up foil to keep them level). Bake for 15–18 minutes until the whites of the eggs are cooked, but the yolks remain slightly runny.

⟫⟫⟫ While the avocados are baking, make the chilli beans. Heat the oil in a large frying pan over a medium heat. Add the spring onions/scallions, red pepper and garlic and fry for 2 minutes until softened. Add the beans, tomatoes and spices and cook for another 5 minutes until softened and heated through. Turn off the heat, season with salt and pepper and stir in half the coriander/cilantro and the lime juice. Serve the chilli beans with the avocado, sprinkled with the remaining coriander/cilantro.

PART-TIME VARIATION

⟫⟫⟫ **Baked avocado with chilli chicken**

Prepare the avocados as instructed, above. Slice **450g/1lb skinless, boneless chicken breasts** and omit the kidney beans. While the avocados are baking, heat **2 tbsp olive oil** in a large frying pan over a medium heat. Add the chicken, **5 sliced spring onions/scallions, 1 chopped, deseeded red pepper** and **2 finely chopped garlic cloves** to the pan and fry for 3 minutes until the chicken starts to colour.

Add **4 chopped, deseeded tomatoes** and **½–1 tsp dried chilli/hot pepper flakes, 2 tsp ground coriander** and **1 tsp ground cumin** and cook for 5 minutes, or until the chicken is cooked. Turn off the heat, season with salt and pepper and stir in most of **1 handful of chopped coriander/cilantro leaves** and the **juice of ½ lime**. Serve the chicken and avocado, sprinkled with the remaining coriander/cilantro.

Chickpea dahl <u>WITH</u> spinach tarka

Canned chickpeas are used here instead of the more usual lentils for a refreshing change. You could, of course, choose dried chickpeas to make the dahl, but this requires a certain amount of forward planning as they'll need soaking overnight and a longer cooking time, which may be stretching it for a weekday meal. If you do opt for dried, halve the quantity of beans. Whichever type of bean you choose, don't skip the spiced spinach tarka as it adds the finishing touch to the whole dish.

>>> Heat the oil in a heavy-based saucepan over a medium-low heat and fry the onion, part-covered, for 8 minutes until very soft. Add 2 of the garlic cloves, the ginger, curry paste and turmeric and cook for 1 minute, stirring.

>>> Pour in the stock and coconut milk and bring to a gentle boil, then turn the heat down, add the chickpeas and simmer, part-covered, for 15 minutes, or until reduced and thickened. Partly crush the chickpeas with a potato masher to thicken the sauce further. Season with salt and pepper.

>>> Meanwhile, to make the spinach tarka, melt the butter in a large sauté pan over a medium-low heat. Add the spices and remaining garlic and cook for 1 minute, then add the spinach and cook, turning it regularly with tongs until evenly wilted, about 2–3 minutes. Serve the spinach tarka on top of the chickpea dahl with a good squeeze of lime juice and a spoonful of yogurt with the chapatis by the side.

SERVES >>> **4**
Preparation time > 20 minutes
Cooking time > 25 minutes

1 tbsp coconut or sunflower oil
1 large onion, finely chopped
4 large garlic cloves, finely chopped
5cm/2in piece of fresh root ginger, peeled and grated
2 heaped tbsp Indian curry paste of choice
2 tsp turmeric
350ml/12fl oz/1½ cups vegetable stock
300ml/10½fl oz/1¼ cups coconut milk
1½ × 400g/14oz cans chickpeas, drained
sea salt and freshly ground black pepper
a good squeeze of lime juice
chapatis and plain yogurt, to serve

>>> **Spinach tarka**
50g/1¾oz/3½ tbsp butter
1 tsp dried chilli/hot pepper flakes
1 tsp cumin seeds
1 tsp nigella seeds
400g/14oz spinach, tough stalks discarded and leaves roughly chopped

Lentil <u>AND</u> apricot pilaf <u>WITH</u> spiced cauliflower

SERVES ⟩⟩⟩ **4**

Preparation time ⟩ 15 minutes
Cooking time ⟩ 20 minutes

500ml/17fl oz/generous 2 cups
    vegetable stock
150g/5½oz/scant 1 cup bulgur wheat
3 tbsp olive oil
1 tbsp ground coriander
1 tbsp ground cumin
1–2 tsp chilli powder, to taste
1 tbsp turmeric
½ head of cauliflower, trimmed and cut
    into florets
1 large onion, chopped
1 red pepper, deseeded
    and chopped
1 courgette/zucchini, diced
2 garlic cloves, finely chopped
60g/2¼oz/scant ½ cup dried apricots,
    roughly chopped
400g/14oz can green lentils, drained
2 large handfuls of chopped coriander/
    cilantro leaves
50g/1¾oz/⅓ cup pistachios, roughly
    chopped
sea salt and freshly ground black
    pepper

This is one of those recipes that can be readily adapted to suit all tastes since both the cauli and the chicken alternative are served in addition to the pilaf. It makes a complete and fulfilling meal, plus any leftovers are ideal for a packed lunch the next day, served at room temperature rather than refrigerator-cold. I also have to mention that cauliflower takes on a new lease of life when coated in spices and roasted until it's just tender but still retains a bit of crunch.

⟩⟩⟩ Preheat the oven to 200°C/400°F/Gas 6. Bring the stock to the boil in a saucepan over a high heat, then stir in the bulgur wheat and return to the boil. Turn the heat to low and simmer for 12–15 minutes, covered, until tender. Drain, if necessary, then return the grains to the pan, cover and leave to stand until needed.

⟩⟩⟩ Meanwhile, mix together half the olive oil and half the spices in a bowl. Add the cauliflower and turn until coated in the spice mix. Season with salt and pepper and tip the cauliflower into a roasting pan and roast for 10–12 minutes until tender.

⟩⟩⟩ Heat the remaining oil in a large non-stick frying pan over a medium heat and fry the onion for 5 minutes until softened. Add the red pepper, courgette/zucchini, garlic, apricots and lentils and cook for another 3–5 minutes, stirring regularly, until softened.

⟩⟩⟩ Add the remaining spices, the cooked bulgur and half the coriander/cilantro to the pan, season with salt and pepper and stir until combined and heated through. Serve topped with the cauliflower and sprinkled with the remaining coriander/cilantro and the pistachios.

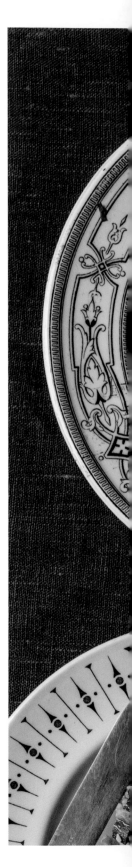

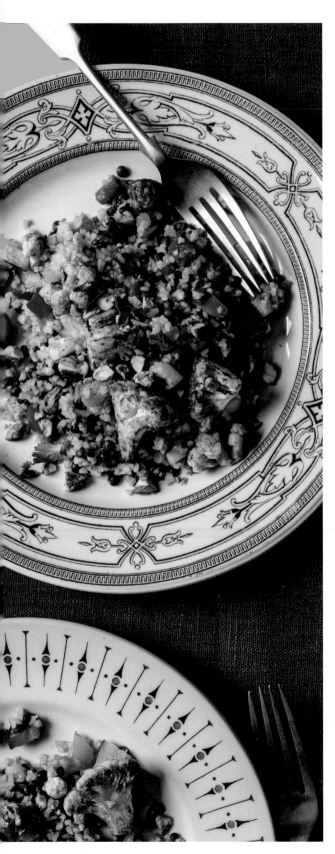

PART-TIME VARIATION

»»» Roasted spiced chicken thighs

Try marinated chicken thighs instead of the spiced roasted cauliflower. First make 3 or 4 cuts in **4–8 chicken thighs**, depending on their size. Mix together **1 tbsp ground coriander, 1 tbsp ground cumin, 2 tsp turmeric** and **1 tbsp paprika**. Season the spice mix and rub it into the chicken until evenly coated. Roast at 200°C/400°F/Gas 6 for 40 minutes, or until cooked through and there is no trace of pink when prodded with a skewer. Serve on top of the pilaf, sprinkled with the coriander/cilantro.

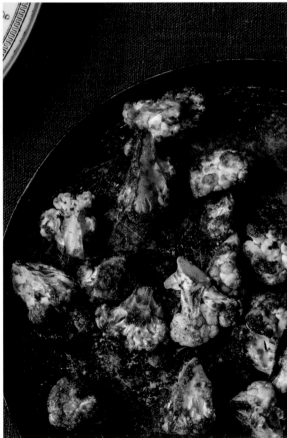

Tomato, olive AND mozzarella rice

SERVES >>> **4**

Preparation time > 15 minutes, plus standing

Cooking time > 40 minutes

2 tbsp extra virgin olive oil, plus extra
   for drizzling
2 large onions, roughly chopped
3 large garlic cloves, finely chopped
225g/8oz/heaped 1 cup paella rice
185ml/6fl oz/¾ cup dry white wine
   (optional)
1 tbsp tomato purée/paste
400g/14oz can chopped tomatoes
600ml/21fl oz/generous 2½ cups
   vegetable stock, plus extra
   if needed
2 heaped tbsp oregano or thyme
   leaves
1–2 tsp hot smoked paprika, to taste
175g/6oz/1¾ cups pitted black olives
125g/4½oz mozzarella cheese, drained,
   patted dry and torn into large bite-
   size pieces
sea salt and freshly ground black
   pepper
3 handfuls of rocket//arugula leaves
   and a good squeeze of lemon juice,
   to serve

There's a blend of cultures here with this paella-cum-risotto dish. It's a great make-and-leave-to-do-its-own-thing kind of meal as the majority of the cooking is done in the oven. It's ready when the tomato rice is tender and the mozzarella oozes into little puddles. I like to top it with spoonfuls of basil pesto or the Caper and Herb Oil (see page 100) or you could add some chorizo and prawns/shrimp.

>>> Preheat the oven to 180°C/350°F/Gas 4. Heat the oil in a large heavy-based, ovenproof casserole pan over a medium-low heat and cook the onions, covered, for 5 minutes until soft but not coloured, stirring occasionally to prevent them sticking. Add the garlic and then the rice. Stir to coat the grains in the oil, then pour in the white wine, if using, and allow to bubble away for 3 minutes until reduced and there is no smell of alcohol.

>>> Add the tomato purée/paste, chopped tomatoes and stock and bring to the boil, stirring occasionally. Stir in the oregano, paprika and half the olives, then season with salt and pepper. Cover the pan with a lid or foil and bake for 20 minutes until the rice is just tender.

>>> Remove from the oven, add a little extra stock if the rice looks too dry, then scatter the mozzarella over the top. Drizzle with a little extra oil and bake for a further 10 minutes, uncovered, or until the mozzarella has melted and is turning golden. Remove from the oven, cover, and leave to stand for 10 minutes. Serve topped with the rocket/arugula, the remaining olives, a drizzle of olive oil and a good squeeze of lemon juice.

PART-TIME VARIATION
>>> Chorizo and prawn/shrimp tomato rice

For a non-vegetarian alternative, add 200g/7oz cubed chorizo to the pan with the onions in the first step and cook for 5 minutes until the chorizo starts to colour. Just before the rice is ready, instead of the mozzarella, fry 300g/10½oz raw peeled king prawns/jumbo shrimp in 2 tbsp olive oil and 1 tsp hot smoked paprika over a medium-high heat for 3 minutes, turning regularly until pink and cooked. Season with salt and pepper and serve on top of the rice with the rocket/arugula, the remaining olives, a drizzle of olive oil and a good squeeze of lemon juice.

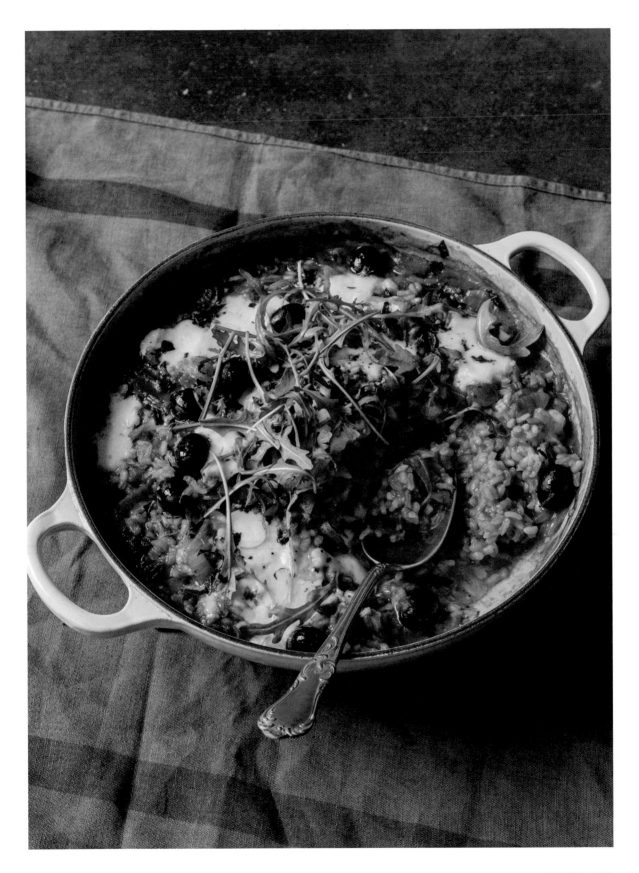

Indonesian stir-fried rice

SERVES ⟩⟩⟩ **4**

Preparation time ⟩ 20 minutes

Cooking time ⟩ 15 minutes

3 tbsp kecap manis (sweet soy sauce)

1 tbsp tomato ketchup

2 tsp turmeric

4 eggs

2 tbsp coconut or sunflower oil, plus
    extra for cooking omelettes

2 banana shallots or 1 onion, chopped

6 spring onions/scallions, sliced, and
    green and white parts separated

125g/4½oz Chinese leaves, shredded

1 large carrot, grated

650g/1lb 7oz/4¾ cups cooked
    cold brown basmati rice (about
    270g/9½oz/heaped 1⅓ cups
    uncooked rice)

2 handfuls of chopped coriander/
    cilantro leaves, to serve

sea salt and freshly ground black
    pepper

⟩⟩⟩ **Peanut paste**

3 large garlic cloves, roughly chopped

3cm/1¼in piece of fresh root ginger,
    peeled and roughly chopped

2 red chillies, deseeded and chopped

60g/2¼oz/generous ½ cup peanuts,
    toasted and roughly chopped
    (see method on page 22)

Based on the classic Indonesian breakfast, *nasi goreng*, this thrifty, complete meal is a great way of using up leftover rice from the night before. If you don't have kecap manis, the Indonesian sweet soy sauce, stir 1 heaped teaspoon soft brown sugar into dark soy sauce instead. For an even speedier meal, use 4 tablespoons crunchy peanut butter instead of the home-made peanut paste. It works well with pork, too.

⟩⟩⟩ To make the peanut paste, blitz the garlic, ginger, chillies and half the peanuts in a mini food processor or grind using a pestle and mortar to a coarse paste.

⟩⟩⟩ Mix together the kecap manis, tomato ketchup and turmeric and leave to one side.

⟩⟩⟩ To make the omelettes, lightly beat 2 of the eggs and season with salt and pepper. Heat a little oil to lightly coat the base of a large non-stick frying pan, add the eggs and tilt the pan to coat the base. Cook for 2 minutes, or until set, then roll up and leave to one side while you cook the second omelette. Cut the omelettes into thin strips, crossways, and leave to one side.

⟩⟩⟩ Heat the remaining oil in a large non-stick wok over a high heat and stir-fry the shallots, the white part of the spring onions/scallions, Chinese leaves and carrot for 4 minutes until softened. Stir in the peanut paste and cook for another 1 minute. Turn the heat down slightly, add the rice and kecap manis mixture and cook, turning constantly, until the rice is thoroughly heated through and piping hot. Gently stir in half the coriander/cilantro and the omelette strips to warm.

⟩⟩⟩ Scatter the reserved green part of the spring onions/scallions and the remaining coriander/cilantro and peanuts over the top and serve straightaway.

PART-TIME VARIATION
⟩⟩⟩ **Shredded pork nasi goreng**

In keeping with the thriftiness of this stir-fried rice dish, stir **250g/9oz shredded leftover roast pork** (or you could use beef or chicken) along with **2 tsp dried shrimp paste** into the rice in place of the omelettes.

For a Korean version, swap the kecap manis for **1 heaped tsp gochujang** and top with the **Easy Kimchi** (see page 165).

Dolcelatte tarts <u>WITH</u> apple nut salad

While it would be something to make your own puff pastry, it's pretty unrealistic for most of us – especially for a weekday meal – and perhaps reassuringly many professional chefs resort to ready-made. Good-quality puff is now readily available and makes a convenient base for savoury or sweet tarts. These Dolcelatte cheese tarts are super simple and come topped with a crisp apple and walnut salad, although you could try the equally easy Goats' Cheese Tarts with Smoked Mackerel Salad on the next page for non-vegetarian friends and family.

⟩⟩⟩ Preheat the oven to 200°C/400°F/Gas 6. Using a small, sharp knife, lightly score a 1cm/½in border around the edge of each pastry rectangle.

⟩⟩⟩ Mash the Dolcelatte in a bowl with the back of a fork, then beat in one of the eggs until smooth and creamy. Spread the mixture over the pastry, within the border, in an even layer. Place the tarts on a large baking sheet. Lightly beat the remaining egg and brush over the border, then season the tarts with pepper and bake for 16–18 minutes until risen and golden.

⟩⟩⟩ While the tarts are cooking, prepare the apple nut salad. Thinly slice the apple into rounds using a mandolin or sharp knife, then halve the slices. ⟩

SERVES ⟩⟩⟩ **4**

Preparation time ⟩ 15 minutes
Cooking time ⟩ 18 minutes

320g/11¼oz sheet ready-rolled puff
   pastry, about 35 × 24cm/
   14 × 9½in, quartered
150g/5½oz Dolcelatte cheese,
   rind removed
2 eggs
sea salt and freshly ground black
   pepper

⟩⟩⟩ **Apple nut salad**
1 eating apple
1 tbsp lemon juice
2 handfuls of rocket/arugula leaves
1 handful of basil leaves, torn
2 tbsp finely snipped chives
1 red chilli, deseeded and diced
4 tsp extra virgin olive oil
2 tbsp walnut pieces, toasted
   (see method on page 22)
2 tbsp sunflower seeds, toasted
   (see method on page 71)
1 tbsp clear honey, for drizzling

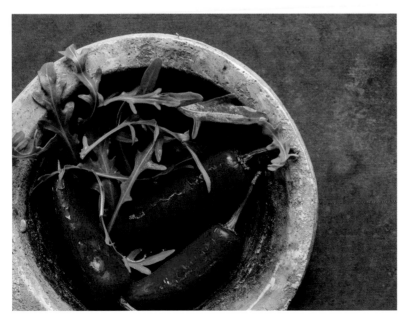

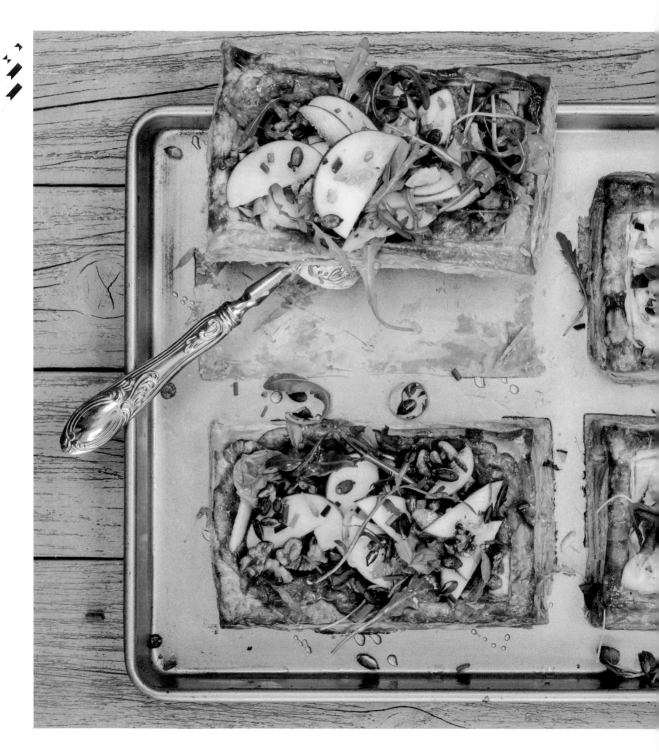

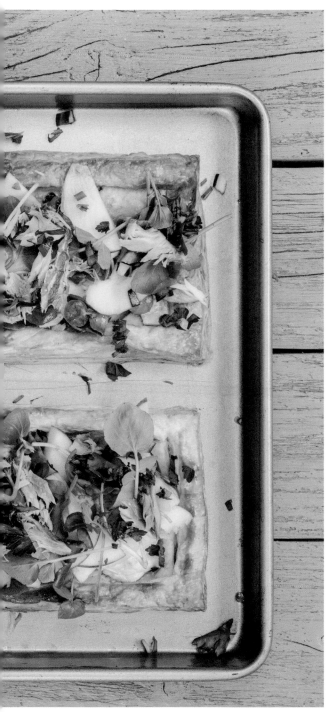

Put the apple in a bowl and toss in the lemon juice to stop it browning. Add the rocket/arugula, herbs, chilli and olive oil to the bowl, season with salt and pepper and toss gently.

>>> Remove the tarts from the oven and leave to cool for a couple of minutes. Pile the apple salad on top of each tart, scatter over the nuts and seeds and drizzle with honey just before serving. (If not serving the tarts straight after baking, hold off topping them with the salad as it will become soggy if left for too long.)

PART-TIME VARIATION
>>> Goats' cheese tarts with smoked mackerel salad

Prepare the cheese tarts as described previously, replacing the Dolcelatte with 150g/5½oz soft, rindless goats' cheese. To make the smoked mackerel salad, thinly slice 1 apple into rounds using a mandolin or sharp knife, then halve each slice. Put the apple in a bowl and toss in 1 tbsp lemon juice to stop it browning. Add 2 handfuls watercress, 1 handful parsley leaves and ¼ diced red onion. Stir in 4 tsp extra virgin olive oil, season and stir until combined. Peel off the skin from 2 smoked mackerel fillets and flake the fish into large pieces. Arrange the mackerel on top of each tart and top with the apple salad.

Quinoa AND borlotti burgers

SERVES ⟫⟫ **4**

Preparation time ⟩ 15 minutes
Cooking time ⟩ 30 minutes

90g/3¼oz/generous ½ cup red quinoa
400g/14oz can borlotti beans, drained
2 spring onions/scallions, finely
    chopped
5 sun-dried tomatoes, finely chopped
½ red pepper, deseeded
    and diced
1 tsp hot smoked paprika
1 tbsp soy sauce
2 tsp dried oregano
flour, for dusting
sunflower oil, for frying
sea salt and freshly ground black
    pepper
rocket/arugula, watercress and spinach
    salad, to serve

⟫⟫ **To finish**

3 tbsp sweet chilli sauce
3 tbsp mayonnaise
4 ciabatta rolls or sesame seed buns,
    split in half and lightly toasted
3 tomatoes, sliced into rounds
2 handfuls of salad leaves
1 avocado, peeled, pitted and diced

Having struggled with the idea of including a veggie burger, mainly due to its old-school vegetarian connotations, this recipe won me over. Quinoa is usually cooked until just tender so it retains a little bite, but here the grain is cooked for slightly longer so it binds readily into a patty with the borlotti beans. The mixture makes four good-size burgers, but you could stretch it to make six, if need be.

⟫⟫ Put the quinoa in a saucepan, cover with water and bring to the boil over a high heat. Turn the heat down and simmer for 20 minutes, covered, until very tender (it should be softer in texture than normal), then drain.

⟫⟫ Meanwhile, mix together the sweet chilli sauce and mayonnaise.

⟫⟫ Tip the cooked quinoa into a food processor with the borlotti beans and process to a coarse paste, leaving some of the beans almost whole. Spoon the mixture into a bowl and stir in the spring onions/scallions, sun-dried tomatoes, red pepper, smoked paprika, soy sauce and oregano. Season with salt and pepper to taste.

⟫⟫ Quarter the mixture and shape each portion into a large burger with floured hands, then lightly dust each burger in flour. Heat enough oil to coat the base of a large non-stick frying pan over a medium heat and fry the burgers for 6–8 minutes, turning once, until golden and crisp. (Alternatively, brush with oil and cook on a baking sheet in the oven preheated to 190°C/375°F/Gas 5 for 25 minutes, turning once, until golden and crisp.)

⟫⟫ To serve, spread each half of the toasted ciabatta rolls with the sweet chilli mayonnaise. Top one half of each roll with the tomato, salad leaves, burger and avocado and then the ciabatta lid. Serve with salad.

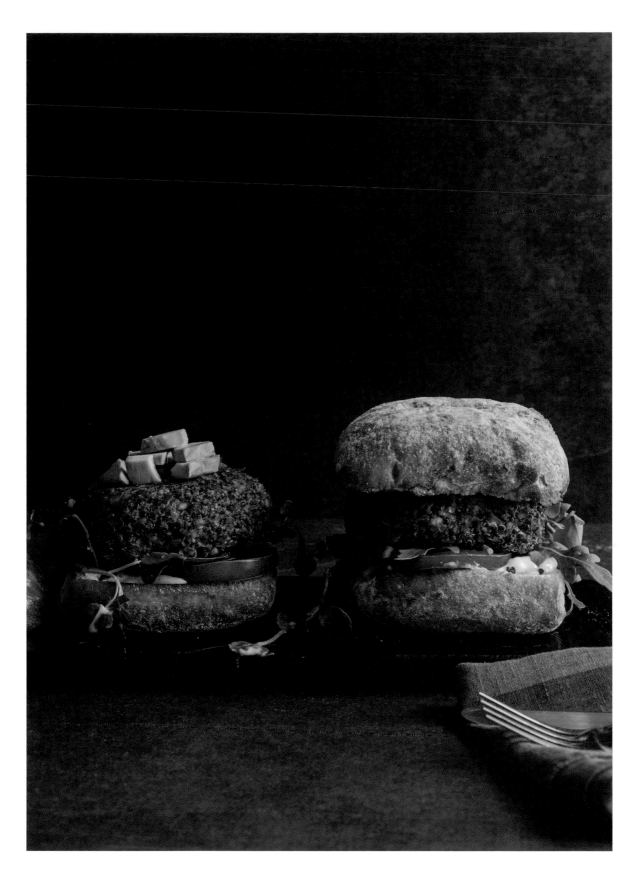

Orecchiette <u>WITH</u> pea <u>AND</u> mint pesto

SERVES ⟩⟩⟩ **4**

Preparation time ⟩ 20 minutes

Cooking time ⟩ 15 minutes

375g/13oz/scant 4 cups dried
orecchiette pasta, or favourite
pasta shape

300g/10½oz/2 cups frozen petit pois

15g/½oz mint leaves

1 large garlic clove, crushed

100ml/3½fl oz/scant ½ cup extra
virgin olive oil, plus extra for frying

20g/¾oz/scant ⅓ cup finely grated
Parmesan cheese, plus extra for
serving

2 tbsp flaked/slivered almonds, toasted
(see method on page 22), plus
extra for serving

4 eggs

sea salt and freshly ground black
pepper

Home-made pesto is my go-to weekday supper as it's infinitely flexible and simple to rustle up when time is short. Here, a classic partnership of pea and mint are blended with toasted almonds, freshly grated Parmesan and extra virgin olive oil and served simply with orecchiette – 'little ears' – pasta. A fried egg on top adds the finishing touch or there is also the option of a salmon fillet.

⟩⟩⟩ Cook the pasta in plenty of boiling salted water, following the pack instructions, until al dente. Drain the pasta, reserving 6 tablespoons of the cooking water.

⟩⟩⟩ Meanwhile, steam the peas for 2–3 minutes until only just tender, then drain and refresh under cold running water. Put three-quarters of the peas in a food processor with the mint, garlic, olive oil, Parmesan and almonds and blitz to a coarse purée, adding a little extra oil if the mixture is too thick, then season with salt and pepper.

⟩⟩⟩ To fry the eggs, heat enough oil to coat the base of a large non-stick frying pan over a medium heat. Crack in the eggs and fry, occasionally spooning the oil over, until the whites are set but the yolks remain runny.

⟩⟩⟩ Meanwhile, return the drained pasta to the cooking pan with the reserved cooking water. Add the reserved cooked peas and enough of the pesto to generously coat the pasta, then toss gently until combined. Transfer the pasta to serving bowls, top with a fried egg and sprinkle with extra Parmesan and almonds. (Any leftover pesto can be spooned into an airtight jar and stored in the refrigerator for up to 1 week. Cover the pesto with a good layer of olive oil to keep it fresh.)

PART-TIME VARIATION

⟩⟩⟩ Orecchiette with pesto and salmon

Place **500g/1lb 2oz thick salmon fillet** in a sauté pan and add enough water to cover. Add **2 bay leaves**, **½ sliced lemon**, **4 peppercorns** and **a few parsley stalks** to flavour the water. Cover and bring to the boil, then turn the heat off and leave the fish to stand in the water until cool. If using a thin fillet, remove from the cooking liquor after 5 minutes. Remove the skin and any bones, flake the fish, season, and serve on top of the pea and mint pesto pasta instead of the egg, Parmesan and almonds.

Caper, crumb AND
lemon linguine

Capers, when fried, turn into moreish crisp, salty nuggets that add a burst of flavour to this pasta dish. It's also a great way of using up bread that is past its best – simply blitz into crumbs and store any leftovers in an airtight container in the freezer, then use straight from frozen.

⟩⟩⟩ Cook the pasta in a large saucepan of boiling salted water, following the pack instructions, until al dente. Drain, reserving 150ml/5fl oz/scant ⅔ cup of the cooking water.

⟩⟩⟩ Meanwhile, heat 1 tablespoon of the oil in a large non-stick frying pan over a medium heat and fry the capers for 6 minutes, turning regularly, until crisp and slightly golden in places. Take care as they can splutter a bit. Remove from the pan with a slotted spoon and leave to one side.

⟩⟩⟩ Add another 2 tablespoons of the oil to the pan and, when hot, add the breadcrumbs and cook for 3–5 minutes until crisp and golden. Stir in the lemon zest then tip into a bowl and leave to one side.

⟩⟩⟩ Wipe the frying pan clean with a crumpled piece of paper towel, then heat the remaining oil over a medium-low heat and cook the tomatoes and garlic for 2 minutes, stirring, until softened. Add the reserved cooking water, the lemon juice and cooked pasta and heat through briefly, tossing until combined. Season with salt and pepper. Serve the pasta sprinkled with the toasted lemon crumbs, capers and parsley.

PART-TIME VARIATION

⟩⟩⟩ Parma ham, crumb and lemon linguine

If capers aren't your thing, try slices of Parma ham instead. Place **8 slices Parma ham** in a large dry, non-stick frying pan over a medium heat and cook for 3–4 minutes, turning once, or until crisp and slightly golden in places. Drain on paper towels and serve broken into large shards on top of the pasta with the toasted lemon crumbs and **1 handful of basil leaves.**

SERVES ⟩⟩⟩ **4**

Preparation time ⟩ 10 minutes
Cooking time ⟩ 15 minutes

375g/13oz dried linguine pasta
4 tbsp extra virgin olive oil
70g/2½oz capers, rinsed and
    patted dry
60g/2¼oz/1 cup day-old fresh
    breadcrumbs
finely grated zest and juice of 1 large
    lemon
6 good-size vine-ripened tomatoes,
    deseeded and diced
2 large garlic cloves, thinly sliced
4 tbsp chopped flat-leaf parsley leaves
sea salt and freshly ground black
    pepper

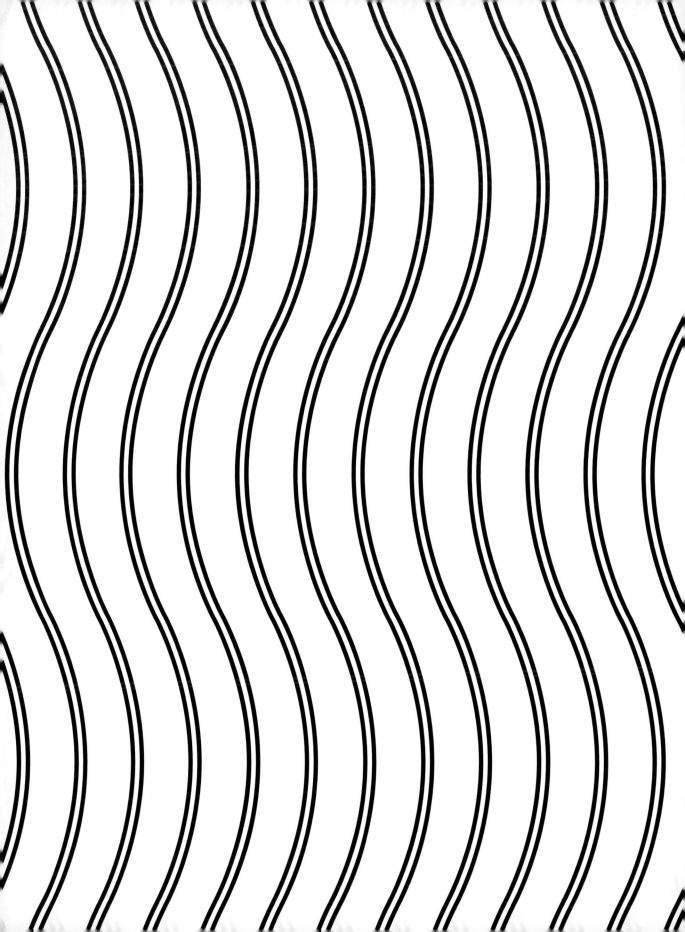

WEEKEND COOKING

Coconut <u>AND</u> kaffir lime broth <u>WITH</u> sweet potato wontons

SERVES ››› **4**

Preparation time › 30 minutes
Cooking time › 40 minutes

400ml/14fl oz/1¾ cups vegetable stock
400g/14oz can coconut milk
1 leek, thinly sliced diagonally
2 red chillies, deseeded and thinly sliced
2.5cm/1in piece of fresh root ginger,
   sliced into rounds
2 lemongrass stalks, outer layer
   removed and stalks bruised
4 fresh kaffir lime leaves, shredded
1 tbsp light soy sauce
1 large handful pea shoots or
   watercress
2 spring onions/scallions, shredded

››› Sweet potato wontons
200g/7oz sweet potatoes, peeled
   and sliced
1.5cm/⅝in piece of fresh root
   ginger, peeled and grated
2 tsp light soy sauce
1 tsp sesame oil
20 square wonton wrappers (for
   steaming), defrosted if frozen
sea salt and freshly ground black
   pepper

Find wonton wrappers for making steamed dumplings in Asian grocers. They're available chilled or frozen and I like to stock up on a few packs, keeping them in the freezer for times when I have a craving for dumplings. These wontons are filled with either a gingery sweet potato purée or crab, for non-vegetarians, and come with a rejuvenating broth.

››› Put the stock, coconut milk, leek, half the chilli, the ginger, lemongrass, lime leaves and soy sauce in a large saucepan and bring to the boil. Turn the heat down and simmer for 10 minutes until reduced. Season with salt and pepper to taste, turn off the heat, cover the pan with a lid, and leave the broth to infuse while you make the wontons.

››› To make the wonton filling, steam the sweet potatoes for 5 minutes, or until tender, then remove the steamer basket from the heat and leave the sweet potatoes to dry. Tip them into a mixing bowl and mash with the back of a fork to a coarse purée, then stir in the ginger, soy sauce and sesame oil. Season with salt and pepper to taste.

››› To fill the wontons, place a teaspoon of the sweet potato mixture in the middle of a wrapper. Lightly dampen the edges of the wrapper with water and fold it over the filling into a triangle. Press the wrapper down around the filling to make a sealed parcel. Fold down the top triangle. Dampen the two corners at the base and bring them together around the middle, overlapping them slightly so they look like they are giving the wonton a hug. Press firmly to join and keep covered with a damp dish towel while you prepare the remaining wontons.

››› Line a large steamer basket with baking paper. Steam the wontons in batches (making sure that they don't touch each other while cooking) for 10–12 minutes until tender.

››› Reheat the coconut broth and remove the lemongrass and ginger. Ladle the broth into large, shallow serving bowls, add the wontons and top with the pea shoots, spring onions/scallions and the remaining chilli.

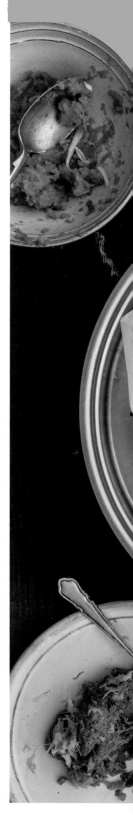

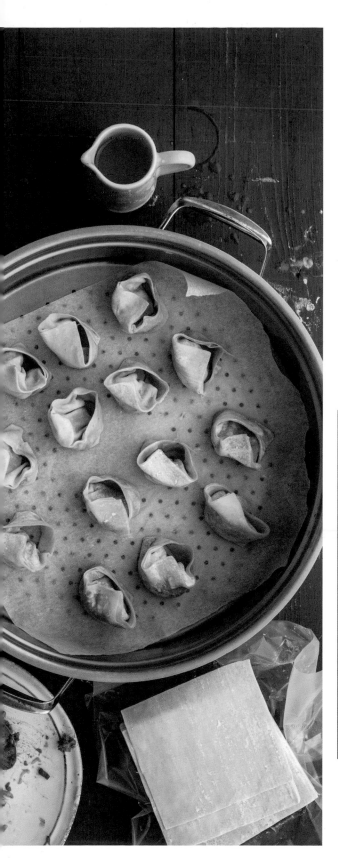

PART-TIME VARIATION

››› Coconut and kaffir lime broth with crab wonton

Prepare the coconut broth as described on the previous page. To make the crab wonton, mix together 150g/5½oz white and brown crab meat, 1 finely chopped spring onion/scallion, 1.5cm/⅝in piece of fresh root ginger, peeled and grated and 1 tsp soy sauce. Fill the wontons with the crab mixture and cook and serve following the instructions described on the previous page.

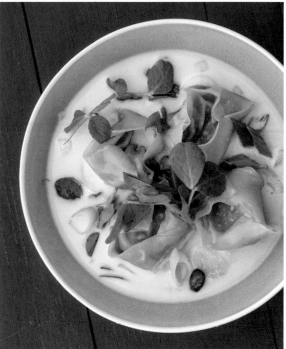

Freekeh, herb AND black olive salad WITH spiced almonds

SERVES ⟩⟩⟩ **4**

Preparation time ⟩ 10 minutes
Cooking time ⟩ 40 minutes

2 large red peppers, halved with stalk
    left, if possible, and deseeded
140g/5oz/heaped ¾ cup freekeh,
    quinoa or bulgur wheat
3 large handfuls of chopped flat-leaf
    parsley leaves
3 large handfuls of chopped coriander/
    cilantro leaves
100g/3½oz/1 cup pitted black olives,
    drained and roughly chopped
6 sun-blush tomatoes, drained and
    finely chopped
3 celery stalks, finely chopped
4 spring onions/scallions, finely
    chopped

⟩⟩⟩ **Lemon dressing**
5 tbsp extra virgin olive oil
finely grated zest and juice of
    1 large lemon

⟩⟩⟩ **Spiced almonds**
1 tbsp olive oil, plus extra for brushing
2 tsp hot smoked paprika
70g/2½oz/½ cup blanched almonds
sea salt and freshly ground black
    pepper

Fresh and vibrant, this salad comes in a roasted red pepper shell. It's best served warm or at room temperature, rather than refrigerator-cold, as this allows the flavours of the fresh ingredients to sing through. If you are unfamiliar with freekeh, this green wheat is picked unripe and then toasted to give it a slightly smoky flavour. The high-protein grain can now be found in many large supermarkets and health food shops.

⟩⟩⟩ Preheat the oven to 200°C/400°F/Gas 6. Brush both sides of the peppers with olive oil and place in a roasting pan. Roast for 35–40 minutes, turning once, until softened and starting to blacken in places.

⟩⟩⟩ While the peppers are roasting, prepare the spiced almonds. Mix together the oil and paprika in a bowl, then season with salt and pepper. Add the almonds and turn to coat them in the spiced oil. Tip the almonds into a baking pan, spread them out in an even layer and roast in the bottom of the oven below the peppers for 10 minutes, turning once, or until they start to turn golden. Remove from the oven and leave to cool.

⟩⟩⟩ Meanwhile, put the freekeh in a pan and cover with water. Bring to the boil, then turn the heat down to low and simmer, covered, for 15 minutes, or until tender. Drain and tip into a serving bowl.

⟩⟩⟩ While the peppers, nuts and freekeh are cooking, mix together the dressing ingredients and season with salt and pepper to taste.

⟩⟩⟩ Add the herbs, olives, sun-blush tomatoes, celery and spring onions/scallions to the freekeh. Pour the dressing over and turn until everything is combined. Taste and adjust the seasoning, adding more salt, pepper and lemon juice, if needed. Spoon the salad into the roasted peppers and serve with the almonds scattered over the top.

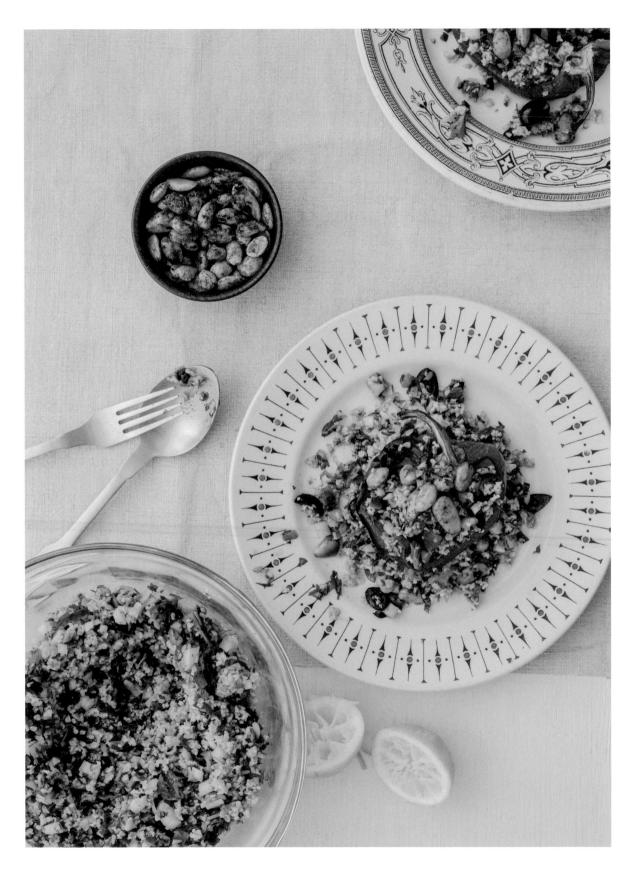

Asparagus AND ginger potstickers

SERVES ⟫⟫ **4**

Preparation time ⟩ 30 minutes
Cooking time ⟩ 6 minutes

20 round wonton wrappers (for
frying), defrosted if frozen
plain/all-purpose flour, for dusting
1 tbsp sunflower oil, plus extra if
needed
1 tbsp finely snipped chives, for
sprinkling

⟫⟫ **Asparagus and ginger filling**
235g/8½oz bunch asparagus, stalks
trimmed and very thinly sliced, tips
halved lengthways
1 spring onion/scallion, finely chopped
2.5cm/1in piece of fresh root ginger,
coarsely grated (no need to peel)
140g/5oz tofu, drained well on paper
towels and coarsely grated
1 tbsp light soy sauce
1 tsp sesame oil
sea salt and freshly ground black
pepper

⟫⟫ **Soy and ginger dipping sauce**
3 tbsp light soy sauce
2 tbsp Chinese black vinegar or
balsamic vinegar
1 tbsp sesame oil
½cm/¼in piece of fresh root ginger,
peeled and finely diced
1 red chilli, deseeded and thinly sliced

'Potsticker' is another name for a Chinese dumpling and this tempting version makes a great precursor to a vegetable stir-fry or can be served as part of dim sum. The great name derives from the way the dumplings are cooked. First they are fried to give a crisp, golden base – take care as they can stick to the pan, hence the name – followed by steaming in a little water or broth. Feel free to try a combination of the filling suggestions, below, depending on personal preference.

⟫⟫ Mix together the ingredients for the dipping sauce, adding just half of the chilli, then leave to one side.

⟫⟫ Reserve the asparagus tips, then mix together the remaining ingredients for the filling in a large bowl and season with a little salt and pepper.

⟫⟫ Place 2 teaspoons of the filling mixture in the centre of a wonton wrapper. Moisten the edge of the wrapper with a little water, fold in half and pleat the edge to seal to make a half moon-shaped dumpling with a flat bottom and rounded top. Place the dumpling on a floured board, cover with a damp dish towel and repeat to make 20 dumplings in total.

⟫⟫ Heat the oil in a large lidded frying pan. Arrange half the dumplings in the pan, flat-side down, and cook for 2 minutes until the base of each dumpling is golden and slightly crisp. Remove from the pan, leave to one side and repeat with the second batch of dumplings, adding more oil, if needed. Return the dumplings to the pan if they fit in an even layer. Add 4 tablespoons water to the pan and scatter over the asparagus tips, immediately cover the pan with a lid and steam for 2 minutes until the liquid is absorbed.

⟫⟫ Serve the dumplings scattered with the asparagus tips, chives and reserved chilli with the dipping sauce in a small bowl by the side.

PART-TIME VARIATION
⟫⟫ Pork and ginger potstickers

To make the potsticker filling, mix together 150g/5½oz minced/ground pork, 1 finely chopped Chinese cabbage leaf, 2.5cm/1in piece of fresh root ginger, grated, 1 finely chopped spring onion/scallion, 1 tbsp light soy sauce and 1 tsp sesame oil in a bowl. Make and cook the dumplings as described above, adding 6 tablespoons water to the pan. Cover with a lid and cook for 6 minutes. Serve scattered with chives and chilli with the dipping sauce.

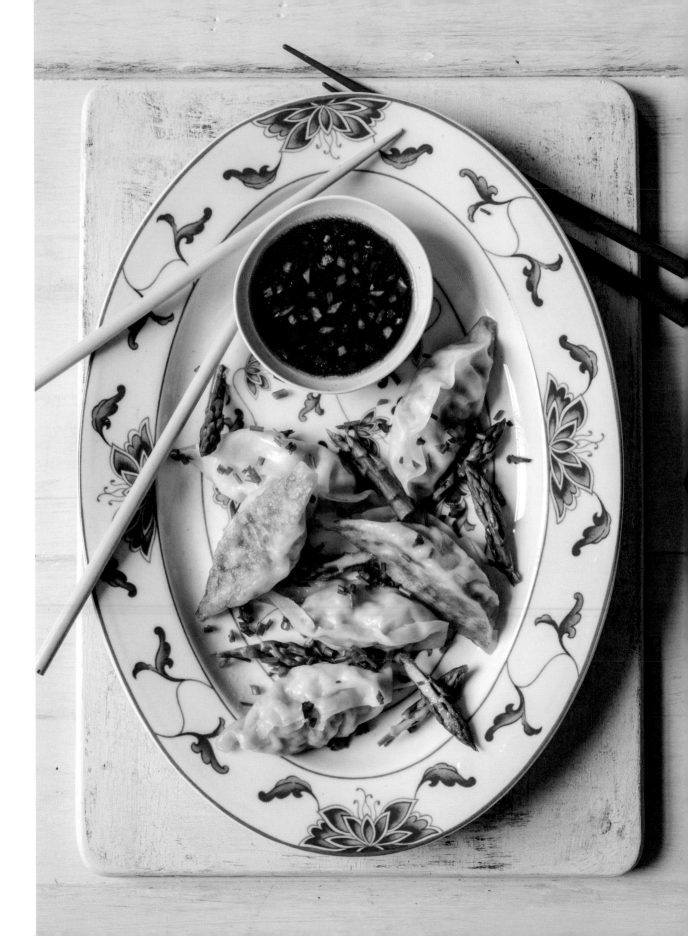

Little cabbages in smoked garlic butter <u>WITH</u> onion cream

SERVES ⟩⟩⟩ **4**

Preparation time ⟩ 20 minutes

Cooking time ⟩ 25 minutes

600g/1lb 5oz new potatoes, scrubbed

70g/2½oz/4½ tbsp butter

280g/10oz Brussels sprouts, trimmed and outer layer discarded

250g/9oz baby leeks, trimmed

200g/7oz baby carrots, trimmed

¼ Savoy cabbage, tough stalks discarded and leaves shredded

3 large smoked garlic cloves, thinly sliced, or 1 tsp smoked garlic powder and 2 garlic cloves

2 tsp chopped rosemary leaves

400g/14oz can butter beans, drained

200ml/7fl oz/scant 1 cup dry white wine or vegetable stock

⟩⟩⟩ **Onion cream**

500g/1lb 2oz onions, cut into thin wedges

1 tsp vegetable bouillon powder

4 tbsp whipping cream

sea salt and freshly ground black pepper

Okay, admittedly 'little cabbages' are Brussels sprouts by another name, yet the intention is not to confuse but hopefully revive interest in the much-maligned brassica. Sprouts are destined to become the 'new kale' and this recipe just goes to show their versatility.

⟩⟩⟩ To make the onion cream, put the onions in a pan and pour in enough water to just cover. Bring to the boil, stir in the bouillon powder, then turn the heat down and simmer for 15 minutes, part-covered, or until the onions are tender. Drain, reserving 100ml/3½fl oz/scant ½ cup of the cooking stock, then return the onions to the pan. Add the cream, half of the stock, season and heat gently until warm. Using a stick/immersion blender, blend the onions to make a thick, smooth, creamy sauce, adding more of the stock if it is too thick. Leave to one side.

⟩⟩⟩ Meanwhile, cook the potatoes in boiling salted water for 12–15 minutes, or until tender. Drain, stir in 2 teaspoons of the butter and crush roughly with a vegetable masher.

⟩⟩⟩ While the onions and potatoes are cooking, steam the sprouts, leeks and carrots for 4 minutes, or until almost tender, then refresh under cold running water. Steam the cabbage for 1–2 minutes, then refresh under cold running water.

⟩⟩⟩ Melt the remaining butter in a large sauté pan over a medium-low heat and add the garlic and rosemary. Cook for 1 minute before adding the beans and wine or stock. Bring to the boil, then turn the heat down and simmer for 3–5 minutes until reduced and there is no aroma of alcohol. Add the steamed vegetables and cook for 1–2 minutes until tender and warmed through. Spoon the crushed potatoes onto plates, top with the vegetables and serve with the onion cream.

PART-TIME VARIATION

⟩⟩⟩ White fish with smoked garlic and onion cream

Prepare the onion cream and crushed potatoes as described above. Omit the sprouts and butter beans and follow the instructions for steaming the leeks, carrots and Savoy cabbage. Melt **1 tbsp butter** in a large sauté pan, add **2 smoked garlic cloves, sliced**, and the steamed vegetables, season, and heat through for a minute. Remove from the pan to a warm dish and cover with foil.

Dust both sides of **4 thick fillets white fish** in **4 tbsp seasoned plain/all purpose flour**. Melt **2 tbsp olive oil** and **1 tbsp butter** in the pan over a medium heat and fry the fish for 5 minutes, turning once, or until golden. Serve the fish and vegetables on top of the crushed potatoes with the onion cream.

Aubergine polpettine

Fried balls of aubergine/eggplant, Parmesan, herbs and breadcrumbs sitting atop a herby tomato sauce makes a simple, comforting dinner. And nothing goes to waste, even the aubergine skin is used – sliced into thin strips and cooked until crisp. To keep fat levels down, steam the aubergines first until meltingly soft.

⟩⟩⟩ Steam the aubergine/eggplant flesh for 15 minutes until very tender. Meanwhile, heat the oil in a large non-stick frying pan and fry the aubergine/eggplant skin in two batches for 2–3 minutes until crisp. Remove with a slotted spoon, drain on paper towels and season with a little salt, then set aside. Leave the frying pan with any remaining oil to one side.

⟩⟩⟩ Put the aubergine/eggplants in a sieve/fine-mesh strainer and press with the back of a spoon to remove any residual water, then tip them into a large bowl and stir in the garlic, Parmesan, breadcrumbs, herbs and eggs. Season well with salt and pepper.

⟩⟩⟩ Take a little of the mixture, about the size of a large walnut, and roll into a ball, then repeat to make about 20 balls in total. Reheat the oil in the frying pan, adding more if needed, over a medium heat. Cook the aubergine/eggplant polpettine in batches for 6–8 minutes, turning occasionally, until golden and starting to crisp all over. Drain on paper towels.

⟩⟩⟩ Heat the tomato basil sauce in a large pan, then transfer the polpettine to the pan and warm through. Serve sprinkled with extra oregano, if you have used fresh, and Parmesan, topped with a heap of crisp aubergine/eggplant skin.

SERVES ⟩⟩⟩ 4
Preparation time ⟩ 20 minutes
Cooking time ⟩ 35 minutes

2 aubergines/eggplants, peeled using a vegetable peeler, flesh diced, and skin cut into long, thin strips
6 tbsp olive oil, plus extra if needed
3 large garlic cloves, finely chopped
80g/2¾oz/1¼ cups finely grated Parmesan cheese, plus extra for serving
180g/6½oz/3 cups day-old fresh breadcrumbs
1 tbsp oregano leaves, plus extra for serving, or 1½ tsp dried
1 tbsp thyme leaves or 1½ tsp dried
2 eggs, lightly beaten
sea salt and freshly ground black pepper
1 recipe quantity Tomato Basil Sauce (see page 200), to serve

Potato pakora burgers

SERVES ⟫⟫⟫ **4**

Preparation time ⟩ 20 minutes

Cooking time ⟩ 25 minutes

480g/1lb 1oz white potatoes, peeled
   and quartered

1½ tsp turmeric

6 spring onions/scallions, finely
   chopped

1 long red chilli, deseeded and finely
   chopped

2 tsp nigella seeds

1 tsp sea salt

2.5cm/1in piece of fresh root ginger,
   peeled and grated

1½ tbsp butter

sunflower oil, for frying

freshly ground black pepper

⟫⟫⟫ Chickpea batter

80g/2¾oz/¾ cup gram/chickpea/
   besan flour

½ tsp sea salt

2 tbsp milk

⟫⟫⟫ To serve

4 small naan breads

4 tbsp Tamarind and Date Chutney
   (see page 67)

4 tomatoes, sliced

1 small red onion, sliced

1 recipe quantity Mint Raita, (see
   page 86), adding 2.5cm/1in piece
   of cucumber, diced

An Indian twist on the regular veggie burger, these spiced potato patties are coated in a gram flour batter and cooked until the outside is crisp and golden. You could make the pre-battered potato patties a few hours ahead of serving, if convenient.

⟫⟫⟫ Put the potatoes in a large pan, pour in enough water to cover and bring to the boil. Add salt and stir in 1 teaspoon of the turmeric and cook for 12–15 minutes until tender.

⟫⟫⟫ While the potatoes are cooking, mix together the ingredients for the batter with the remaining turmeric. Whisk in 5–6 tablespoons water to make a smooth, pancake-batter consistency. Leave to rest until needed.

⟫⟫⟫ Drain and return the potatoes to the still-hot pan to dry, then when cool enough to handle, coarsely grate them into a mixing bowl. Stir in the spring onions/scallions, chilli, nigella seeds, salt, ginger and butter, allowing the latter to melt in the heat of the potatoes. Season with pepper and stir until combined, then, using your hands, form the mixture into 4 large patties.

⟫⟫⟫ Heat enough oil in a pan to deep-fry the pakora burgers. The oil is hot enough when a cube of bread turns golden in 30 seconds. Dip each patty into the batter mixture until thickly coated, then fry two at a time for 1½–2 minutes, or until golden all over. Drain on paper towels and keep warm in a low oven while you cook the remaining pakora burgers. Wrap the naan in foil and warm them in the oven at the same time.

⟫⟫⟫ To serve, top each naan with a spoonful of the chutney. Place a few slices of tomato on top before adding the pakora burger, red onion and a spoonful of the mint raita.

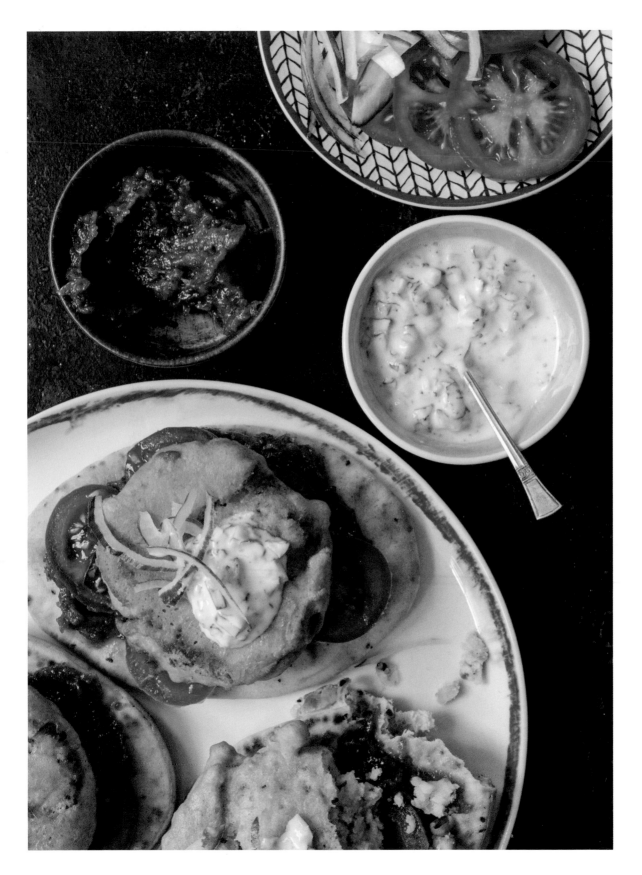

Brazilian sweet potato AND red pepper curry

SERVES ⟩⟩⟩ **4**

Preparation time ⟩ 15 minutes
Cooking time ⟩ 35 minutes

2 tbsp coconut or sunflower oil

1 large onion, coarsely grated

3 garlic cloves, coarsely grated

4cm/1½in piece of fresh root ginger,
    peeled and finely chopped

1 large red pepper, deseeded
    and chopped

2 red chillies, deseeded and finely
    chopped

400g/14oz can coconut milk

250ml/9fl oz/generous 1 cup
    vegetable stock

2 tbsp tomato purée/paste

1 tsp turmeric

1 tsp cayenne pepper

550g/1lb 4oz sweet potatoes, peeled
    and cut into large bite-size chunks

1 large courgette/zucchini, quartered
    lengthways and cut into chunks

85g/3oz kale, tough stalks removed
    and finely chopped

2 tomatoes, deseeded and diced

1 large handful of chopped coriander/
    cilantro leaves

sea salt and freshly ground black
    pepper

black rice or brown basmati rice,
    to serve

1 lime, cut into wedges, to serve

This has become one of my favourite curries, as much for its simplicity as its great colour and flavour. It comes with black rice with its slightly nutty taste and firm texture, which works so well with the creaminess of the coconut sauce as well as adding a wonderful contrast in colour. The prawn/shrimp variation has similar flavourings, but comes without the sweet potatoes and courgettes/zucchini.

⟩⟩⟩ Heat the oil in a large saucepan over a medium heat and fry the onion for 5 minutes, stirring often, until softened. Turn the heat down slightly, add the garlic, ginger, red pepper and half the chillies and cook for another 3 minutes, stirring often.

⟩⟩⟩ Pour in the coconut milk and stock and bring to the boil. Turn the heat down slightly, stir in the tomato purée/paste, turmeric and cayenne and simmer, stirring occasionally, for 5 minutes. Add the sweet potatoes, return to a gentle boil and cook for 10 minutes, part-covered, until almost tender.

⟩⟩⟩ Add the courgette/zucchini, kale and tomatoes and simmer for another 3–5 minutes, part-covered, or until the vegetables are cooked through. Stir the curry occasionally to prevent it sticking and add a splash more stock or water, if the sauce looks dry. Season with salt and pepper, sprinkle with coriander/cilantro and the remaining chilli and serve with rice and a wedge of lime by the side.

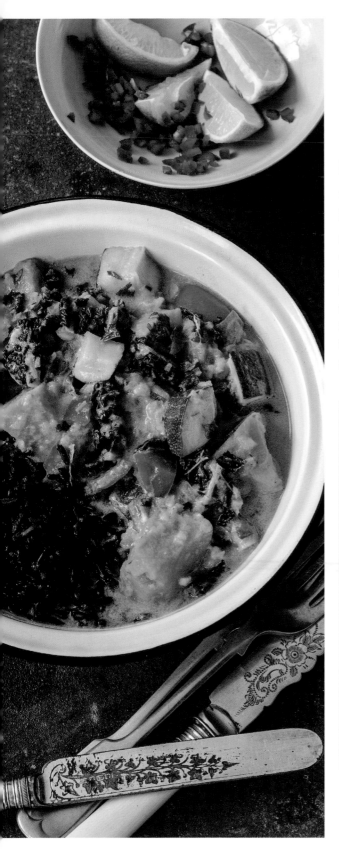

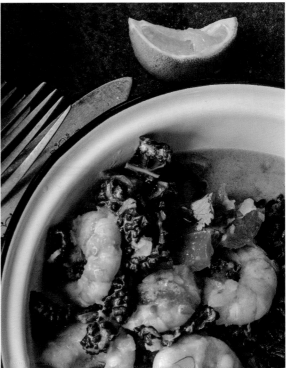

PART-TIME VARIATION

⟩⟩⟩ Prawn/shrimp and red pepper curry

Replace the sweet potato and courgette/zucchini with 400g/14oz peeled large raw prawns/jumbo shrimp. Reduce the quantity of stock to 200ml/7fl oz/scant 1 cup and use fish stock in place of vegetable. Add the prawns/shrimp to the pan at the same time as the kale and tomatoes (omitting the courgette/zucchini) and cook for 3–5 minutes until the prawns/shrimp turn pink. Serve as described on the previous page.

Beetroot tarts WITH Scandinavian flavours

MAKES ⟩⟩⟩ **6 TARTS**

Preparation time ⟩ 45 minutes
Cooking time ⟩ 30 minutes

⟩⟩⟩ Rye pastry

125g/4½oz/1 cup plain/all-purpose
   flour
50g/1¾oz/½ cup rye flour
½ tsp sea salt, plus extra for the pickle
90g/3¼oz/6 tbsp chilled butter, cut into
   small pieces, plus extra for greasing
1 tbsp sour cream

⟩⟩⟩ Beetroot/beet filling

1 tsp caraway seeds
300g/10½oz cooked beetroot/beets
   (not in vinegar), patted dry
juice of ½ lemon
6 tbsp sour cream
yolks from 2 large hard-boiled eggs,
   crumbled
freshly ground black pepper

⟩⟩⟩ Cucumber and fennel pickle

1 small cucumber, halved crossways
   and sliced into long, thin strips,
   seeds discarded
1 fennel bulb, sliced into long, thin
   strips, fronds reserved
2 tbsp caster/granulated sugar
4 tbsp white wine vinegar
1 tbsp chopped dill, plus extra for
   serving

This was a bit of an experiment. I love the fresh, vibrant quality of Scandinavian cooking and wanted to capture an essence of this with these beetroot/beet tarts, which come with a fresh cucumber and fennel pickle. The rye pastry can be replaced with 375g/13oz ready-made shortcrust, if you prefer.

⟩⟩⟩ To make the rye pastry, sift both types of flour and the salt into a mixing bowl. Rub in the butter with your fingertips until you have a fine breadcrumb texture. Stir in the 1 tablespoon of sour cream and enough water to make a ball of dough, about 2 tablespoons. Wrap the dough in cling film/plastic wrap and chill for 30 minutes.

⟩⟩⟩ Meanwhile, make the pickle. Put the cucumber and fennel in a sieve/fine mesh strainer suspended over a bowl, douse in plenty of salt and leave for 30 minutes.

⟩⟩⟩ To make the filling for the tarts, toast the caraway seeds in a dry frying pan for 2 minutes, or until they smell aromatic. Grind the seeds to a powder in a pestle and mortar. Using a stick/immersion blender, blend the beetroot/beets to a purée then add a squeeze of lemon juice, the ground caraway and season with salt and pepper. Leave to one side.

⟩⟩⟩ Preheat the oven to 180°C/350°F/Gas 4. Grease 6 × 10cm/4in fluted tart pans with butter. Roll out the pastry and use to line the prepared tart pans, then place them on a baking sheet. Prick the pastry bases, line with baking paper and beans and bake blind for 15 minutes until the edges of the pastry start to colour. Remove the beans and paper and return to the oven for another 15 minutes, or until cooked.

⟩⟩⟩ While the pastry cases are cooking, finish making the pickle. Rinse the cucumber and fennel, drain and pat dry in a clean dish towel. Mix the sugar into the vinegar until dissolved, add the vegetables and dill and stir until combined.

⟩⟩⟩ Spoon the puréed beetroot/beets into the cooked pastry cases, top with a spoonful of sour cream, a squeeze of lemon juice and the crumbled egg yolks. Serve the tarts sprinkled with fennel fronds and/or dill and with the pickle.

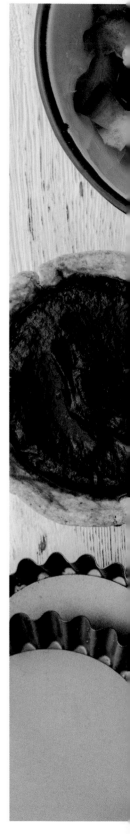

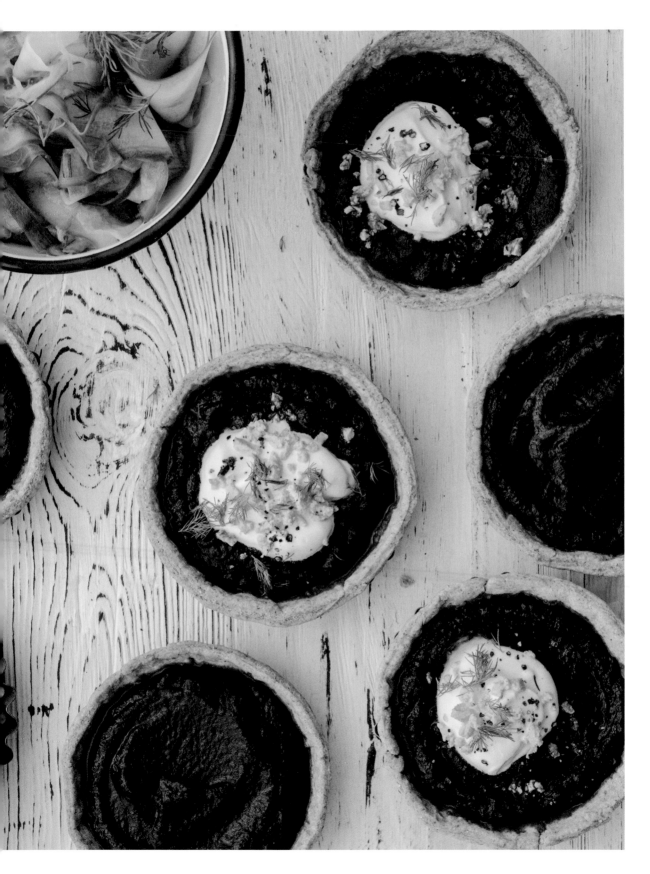

Shallot tarte tatin

SERVES ⟩⟩⟩ **4–6**

Preparation time ⟩ 15 minutes, plus resting

Cooking time ⟩ 40 minutes

40g/1½oz/2½ tbsp butter, plus extra
   for greasing
2 tbsp olive oil
450g/1lb echalions or banana shallots,
   peeled and halved lengthways
2 tbsp balsamic vinegar
2 tsp soft light brown sugar
1 tbsp thyme leaves, plus extra
   sprigs for serving
400g/14oz puff pastry
flour, for dusting
sea salt and freshly ground black
   pepper
peppery green salad, to serve

A fresh, peppery green salad is all you need with this caramelized shallot tarte tatin to make a delicious light meal. For a more substantial tatin, you could scatter a crumbled piquant blue cheese and toasted chopped hazelnuts over the top. Echalion, or banana shallots, are actually a cross between an onion and a shallot with an attractive elongated shape, and are conveniently easy to peel.

⟩⟩⟩ Preheat the oven to 200°C/400°F/Gas 6. Heat the butter and oil in a large frying pan over a medium heat. Add the echalions and cook for 8–10 minutes, turning occasionally, until tender and light golden. Remove and discard (or save for another dish) the outer layer of each echalion if it starts to peel away during cooking or becomes too dark. Stir in the balsamic vinegar and sugar and cook for 1 minute until the sauce has reduced and is slightly syrupy.

⟩⟩⟩ Lightly grease a 23cm/9in shallow non-stick cake pan and line the base with baking paper. Arrange the echalions in a single even layer in the pan, pour any syrupy sauce left in the frying pan over and scatter with half the thyme. Season with salt and pepper.

⟩⟩⟩ Roll the pastry out on a lightly floured work surface to a 26cm/10½in circle. Place on top of the echalions, tucking the edge of the pastry down the sides of the pan. Bake for 30 minutes until the pastry is risen and golden. Leave in the pan for 10 minutes, then invert onto a serving plate. Peel away the baking paper, scatter over the remaining thyme and top with a few extra sprigs. Cut into wedges and serve with a peppery green salad.

Roasted pepper AND
pine nut pissaladière

This classic Provençal 'pizza' is topped with a Mediterranean-inspired combination of roasted peppers, lemon thyme, black olives and toasted pine nuts. For a speedy alternative, you could use roasted peppers from a jar or, for pescatarians, the anchovy variation on the next page with a sheet of puff pastry as a base – either way, it is delicious served simply with a tomato and basil salad.

⟩⟩⟩ To make the base, mix together the yeast, sugar and 1 tablespoon of lukewarm water in a small bowl and leave until slightly frothy, about 10 minutes.

⟩⟩⟩ Put the flour and salt in a large mixing bowl, stir and make a well in the centre, then add the egg, 1 tablespoon of the oil, 5 tablespoons of lukewarm water and the yeast mixture. Mix until the dough comes together, adding a little more lukewarm water if the mixture is too dry or a little more flour, if too wet.

⟩⟩⟩ Turn the dough out onto a lightly floured work surface and knead for 5 minutes until it comes together into a smooth and elastic ball. Put the dough in a lightly oiled bowl, cover with cling film/plastic wrap, and leave in a warm place while you prepare the onions.

⟩⟩⟩ Preheat the grill/broiler to high. Heat the remaining oil in a large non-stick frying pan over a medium heat. Add the onions and turn the heat down slightly. ⟩

SERVES ⟩⟩⟩ **4–6**
Preparation time ⟩ 30 minutes, plus proving
Cooking time ⟩ 45 minutes

1 heaped tsp instant dried yeast
½ tsp caster/granulated sugar
250g/9oz/2 cups strong white flour, plus extra for dusting
1 tsp salt
1 egg, beaten
3 tbsp extra virgin olive oil, plus extra for greasing and drizzling
6 onions (about 800g/1lb 12oz total weight), halved and thinly sliced
3 garlic cloves, thinly sliced
2 large red peppers, halved, deseeded and cut into long wedges
1 handful of pitted black olives
3 tbsp lemon thyme leaves
2 tbsp pine nuts, toasted (see method on page 22)
freshly ground black pepper

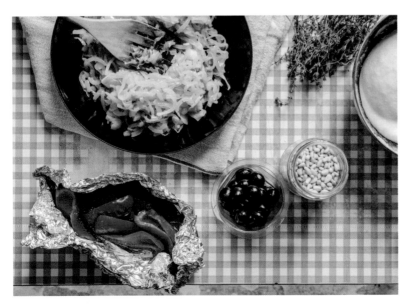

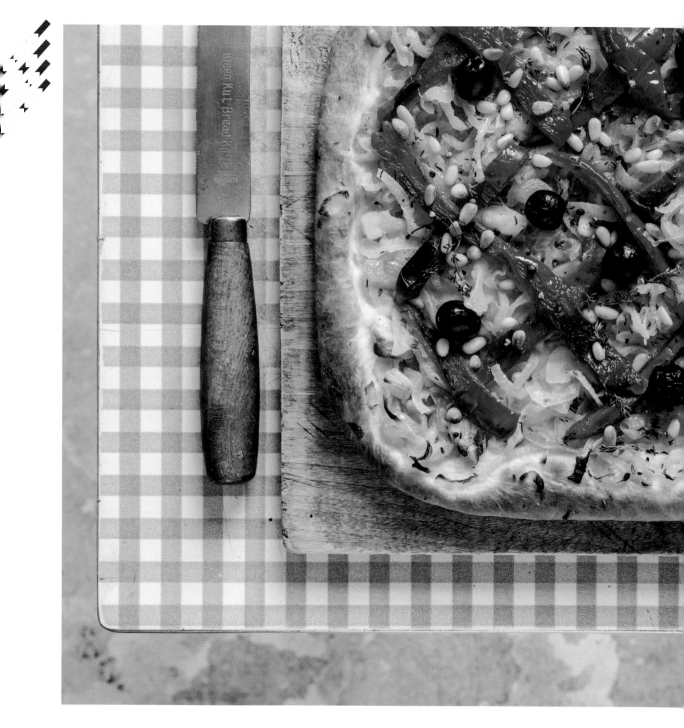

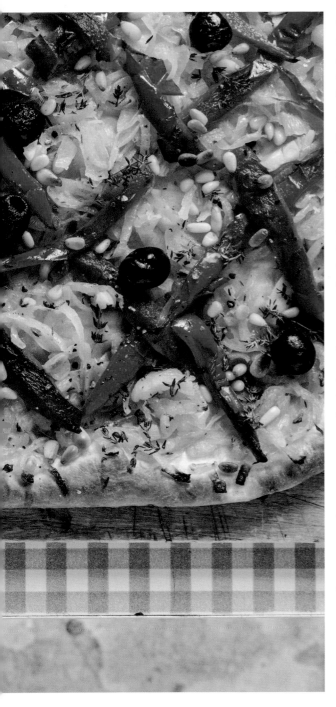

Cook for 20 minutes, covered and stirring occasionally, until softened but not coloured. Remove the lid of the pan 5 minutes before the end of the cooking time to cook off any liquid. Add the garlic and cook for 1 minute until softened. Leave to cool slightly.

››› Meanwhile, brush both sides of the red peppers with oil and line the grill/broiler pan with foil. Grill/broil the peppers for 15 minutes, turning once, until tender and blackened in places. Put the peppers in a small plastic bag and leave for 5 minutes to make them easier to peel.

››› Lightly oil a large shallow baking pan, about 26 × 40cm/10½ × 16in. Roll out the dough and use to line the baking pan, pressing the dough slightly up at the edge to make a lip. Leave the base to prove for 20 minutes while you preheat the oven to 220°C/425°F/Gas 7.

››› Spoon the onion mixture evenly on top of the base, leaving a border. Peel the peppers, cut into long, thin strips and arrange on top in a criss-cross pattern. Season with pepper and top with the olives and half of the thyme. Bake for 20–25 minutes until the base is cooked and golden. Sprinkle with the remaining thyme and pine nuts and serve warm, cut into wedges.

PART-TIME VARIATION
››› Anchovy and basil pissaladière

Try swapping the red pepper, lemon thyme and pine nuts with **marinated anchovy fillets** in oil or salted ones, depending on your preference. Soak the salted ones first in a little milk for a few minutes to curb the excess saltiness, then rinse and pat dry. Arrange **60g/2¼oz anchovy fillets** on top of the onion mixture following the instructions described above, then sprinkle with basil after baking.

Porcini risotto <u>WITH</u> cavolo nero <u>AND</u> cobnuts

SERVES ⟩⟩⟩ **4**

Preparation time ⟩ 15 minutes, plus soaking

Cooking time ⟩ 40 minutes

30g/1oz/1 cup dried porcini mushrooms

2 tbsp olive oil

1 tbsp butter

1 large onion, finely chopped

200g/7oz chestnut/cremini mushrooms, sliced

320g/11¼oz/1¾ cups risotto rice

175ml/6fl oz/¾ cup dry white wine (optional)

2 tbsp thyme leaves

1 litre/35fl oz/4⅓ cups hot porcini stock or vegetable stock, plus extra if needed

200g/7oz cavolo nero, tough stalks discarded, leaves sliced

juice of ½ lemon and 1 tsp grated lemon zest

plenty of freshly grated Parmesan cheese, to serve (optional)

60g/2oz/½ cup shelled cobnuts or blanched hazelnuts, toasted and roughly chopped (see method on page 22)

sea salt and freshly ground black pepper

Just a handful of dried porcini mushrooms is enough to add a wonderfully rich, savoury flavour to this risotto. The cobnuts complement the earthiness of the porcini as well as adding a bit of crunch, contrasting with the creaminess of the risotto rice. Cobnuts are cultivated hazelnuts and can be bought fresh in their husks and shells in late summer and dried later on in the year. If you have difficulty in finding them, opt for hazelnuts instead. This risotto also works with pearl barley. Simply rinse and soak the barley for 1 hour, then cook for 45 minutes until the grain is tender and creamy.

⟩⟩⟩ Soak the dried porcini in 200ml/7fl oz/scant 1 cup just-boiled water for 20 minutes, then drain, reserving the soaking liquid. Squeeze out any liquid in the porcini, then roughly chop.

⟩⟩⟩ Meanwhile, heat half the oil and the butter in a large heavy-based saucepan over a medium-low heat. Add the onion and cook for 5 minutes, part-covered and stirring occasionally, until softened. Stir in the soaked porcini and chestnut/cremini mushrooms and sauté for another 5 minutes until tender.

⟩⟩⟩ Stir in the rice until coated in the onion mixture, then pour in the wine, if using. Let the wine bubble away until reduced and there is no aroma of alcohol and then strain in the porcini soaking liquid. Stir in the thyme and start to add the hot stock, a ladleful at a time, stirring constantly and only adding the next ladleful when the previous one has been absorbed by the rice. Continue cooking for about 25 minutes, or until the rice is creamy with a slight bite and the texture of the risotto is slightly soupy. Season with salt and pepper, cover with a lid, and leave to stand while you cook the cavolo nero.

⟩⟩⟩ Heat the remaining oil in a large sauté pan over a medium-low heat and sauté the cavolo nero for 2–3 minutes until tender. Add the lemon juice and zest, season with salt and pepper and cook for another minute. Serve on top of the risotto with grated Parmesan, if using, and the cobnuts scattered over.

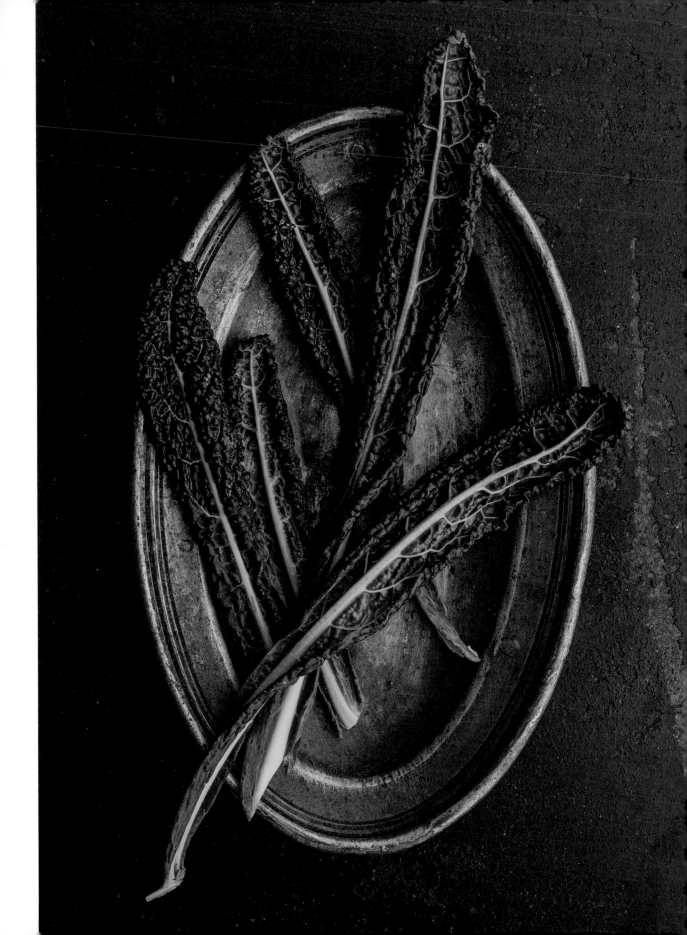

Turnip, olive AND preserved lemon tagine

SERVES ⟩⟩⟩ **4**

Preparation time ⟩ 15 minutes

Cooking time ⟩ 40 minutes

2 tbsp olive oil

2 onions, sliced

3 garlic cloves, thinly sliced

3 turnips, peeled and cut into
   bite-size cubes

2 large carrots, halved lengthways
   and sliced

200g/7oz new potatoes, cut into
   bite-size cubes

500ml/17fl oz/generous 2 cups
   vegetable stock

85g/3oz/heaped ¾ cup green olives

400g/14oz can chickpeas, drained

1 tsp ground cumin

2 tsp ground coriander

2 tsp turmeric

½ tsp ground ginger

½ tsp dried chilli/hot pepper flakes

½ cinnamon stick

½ recipe quantity of Cheat's Preserved
   Lemons (see page 165) and 2 tbsp
   lemon juice, or the shop-bought
   equivalent, flesh discarded and skin
   finely chopped and 2 tbsp juice
   from the jar

1 handful of chopped coriander/
   cilantro leaves

sea salt and freshly ground black
   pepper

couscous, to serve

Turnip is a much underrated and underused vegetable, yet its slightly 'radishy' flavour and crisp texture lends itself to both raw and cooked dishes. Try grating it into slaws or pickles, combining with celeriac or potato to make an alternative mash, or slow cooking until melt-in-the-mouth tender. Don't be put off by the long list of ingredients, this tagine is very much a bung-it-all-in-and-let-it-cook type of dish.

⟩⟩⟩ Heat the oil in a large heavy-based casserole over a medium heat. Add the onions and cook for 5 minutes until softened, then stir in the garlic, turnips, carrots and new potatoes.

⟩⟩⟩ Pour in the stock and add the olives, chickpeas and spices. Bring to the boil, stir well, then turn the heat down to low and simmer for 30 minutes, covered, until the vegetables are tender when prodded with a fork. Stir the tagine occasionally to prevent it sticking and only part-cover the pan if you find you need to cook off some of the liquid.

⟩⟩⟩ Add the preserved lemons and juice, season with salt and pepper, and cook for another 5 minutes, uncovered, or until the sauce has reduced and thickened. Serve sprinkled with the coriander/cilantro and with couscous.

PART-TIME VARIATION

⟩⟩⟩ Chicken and preserved lemon tagine

This variation replaces some of the vegetables in the original recipe with chicken thighs. Brown **6 skinless chicken thighs** in **1 tbsp olive oil** for 5 minutes, turning once, then remove them from the casserole. Add another **1 tbsp olive oil** and cook the vegetables (reduce to **2 turnips** and **2 carrots** and omit the potatoes). Just before adding **420ml/14½fl oz/1¾ cups chicken stock**, omit the chickpeas and return the chicken to the casserole with the spices and continue to cook the tagine as described, above, but extending the main cooking time to 50 minutes instead of 30 minutes.

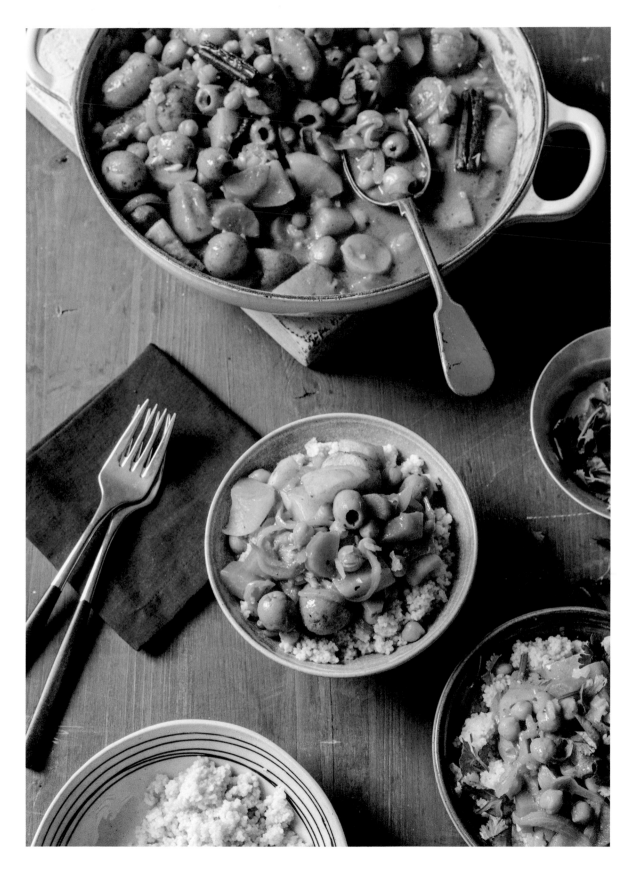

Chipotle black beans
<u>WITH</u> corn flatbreads

SERVES ⟩⟩⟩ **4–6**

Preparation time ⟩ 20 minutes

Cooking time ⟩ 25 minutes

2 tbsp olive oil

1 large onion, chopped

1 large red pepper, deseeded
and chopped

2 large garlic cloves, chopped

1 tsp cumin seeds

1 large corn-on-the-cob, kernels only

2 x 400g/14oz cans black beans
(not drained)

4 tomatoes, deseeded and diced

4 tbsp tomato ketchup

1 tbsp balsamic vinegar

1 tsp clear honey

1 tbsp chipotle paste or 2 tsp hot
smoked paprika

½–1 tsp dried chilli/hot pepper flakes

2 large handfuls of chopped coriander/
cilantro leaves

sea salt and freshly ground black
pepper

⟩⟩⟩ To serve

4 Corn Flatbreads (see page 84)
or corn tortillas, warmed

2 large handfuls of rocket/arugula
leaves

1 large avocado, pitted, peeled
and sliced

1 small red onion, thinly sliced

2 handfuls grated Monterey Jack
or mature, sharp Cheddar cheese

4 tbsp sour cream or plain yogurt

Great for a weekend dinner with family or friends, the idea is to put the flatbreads, black bean sauce (and/or the Cheat's Pulled Pork) and various accompaniments on the table and just let everyone help themselves. The smoky heat of the chipotle chilli combined with the tomato ketchup, balsamic vinegar and honey makes a rich, barbecue-style sauce for the black beans, which is always a winner with the kids. For convenience, the pork variation also uses similar flavouring ingredients as a marinade. Spoon the beans and/or pork on top of the home-made corn flatbreads, or serve with tortillas, rice or tacos. Both the beans and the pork can be made in advance, if you like – in fact this gives the flavours a chance to develop. The beans can be reheated, but avoid this with the pork.

⟩⟩⟩ Heat the oil in a large heavy-based pan and fry the onion for 7 minutes until softened, then add the red pepper, garlic, cumin and corn and cook for another 2 minutes.

⟩⟩⟩ Stir in the black beans, with any liquid from the can, the tomatoes, ketchup, balsamic vinegar, honey, chipotle paste, chilli/hot pepper flakes and 4 tablespoons water. Bring to the boil, stir in half the coriander/cilantro, then turn the down heat to low and simmer for 15 minutes, part-covered and stirring occasionally, until cooked through and the sauce has reduced and thickened. Add a splash of water if the sauce seems too thick. Season with salt and pepper to taste.

⟩⟩⟩ Serve the bean stew on top of the warmed corn flatbreads, topped with the rocket/arugula, avocado, red onion, cheese and a spoonful of sour cream. Scatter the remaining coriander/cilantro over the top before serving.

PART-TIME VARIATION

››› Cheat's pulled pork

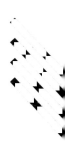

A pork shoulder joint needs cooking for a good 3–4 hours (if not longer) until tender, but this cheat's version of pulled pork uses shoulder steaks and takes a fraction of the time.

Mix together the ingredients for the marinade in a large shallow dish, including 1 tbsp finely ground coffee, 1 tbsp chipotle paste, 1 tbsp honey, 3 tbsp tomato ketchup, 2 large crushed garlic cloves, ½ tsp dried chilli/hot pepper flakes, 1 tsp dried oregano and 1 tsp ground cumin.

Season the marinade with salt and pepper, add **4 thick pork shoulder steaks (about 800g/1lb 12oz total weight)** and turn until coated. Leave to marinate, covered, in the refrigerator for at least 1 hour.

Preheat the oven to 170°C/325°F/Gas 3. Heat **2 tbsp olive oil** in a large frying pan over a medium heat and cook the pork in two batches for 5 minutes, turning once, until browned all over. Spoon any leftover marinade into a small saucepan and add the juices from the frying pan.

Put the pork in a large roasting pan and roast for 30 minutes. Pour off any juices into the saucepan, turn the pork and cook for another 30 minutes, or until tender and slightly blackened around the edges. Cover the pan with foil and leave to rest for 15 minutes.

Meanwhile, heat **1 tbsp olive oil** in a large heavy-based frying pan over a medium heat and fry **1 large sliced onion** for 7 minutes until softened, then add **1 large chopped red pepper**, **2 large chopped garlic cloves**, **1 tsp ground cumin** and the kernels from **1 large corn-on-the-cob** and cook for another 2 minutes.

Heat the pork juices in the pan to make a sauce. Shred the pork with 2 forks and combine with the onion and pepper mixture. Serve on warmed corn flatbreads with the pan juices, rocket/arugula, avocado, red onion, a spoonful of sour cream or yogurt and coriander/cilantro leaves.

Moroccan harira

SERVES ⟩⟩⟩ **6**

Preparation time ⟩ 20 minutes
Cooking time ⟩ 35 minutes

2 large onions, chopped
2 celery stalks, sliced
2 large carrots, halved lengthways
    and sliced
100g/3½oz/½ cup green or Puy lentils
1 tsp turmeric
½ tsp ground cinnamon
2 tsp ground ginger
1 tbsp ground coriander
2 handfuls of coriander/cilantro sprigs,
    leaves chopped and stalks sliced
2 handfuls of flat-leaf parsley sprigs,
    leaves chopped and stalks sliced
400g/14oz can chickpeas, drained
100g/3½oz/½ cup basmati rice
2 tbsp vegetable bouillon powder
4 handfuls of cavolo nero or kale,
    tough stalks discarded and leaves
    torn into bite-size pieces
10 baby plum tomatoes, quartered
50g/1¾oz/3½ tbsp butter
sea salt and freshly ground black
    pepper
crusty bread and lemon wedges,
    to serve

Hugely popular in Morocco, this hearty, fragrant soup-cum-stew is traditionally served during the period of Ramadan to break the fast at sunset. There are many variations of this dish, but all have one thing in common and that is an aromatic blend of herbs and spices.

⟩⟩⟩ Put the onions in a large heavy-based saucepan with the celery, carrots, lentils, spices, coriander/cilantro stalks, parsley stalks and 2 litres/70fl oz/ 8¾ cups water and bring to the boil. Turn the heat down slightly and simmer for 15 minutes, part-covered. Stir in the chickpeas and cook for another 15 minutes, or until the lentils are tender.

⟩⟩⟩ Meanwhile, put the rice in a separate pan and cover with plenty of cold water. Bring to the boil, then turn the heat down and cook, part-covered, for 12 minutes, or until tender. Drain the rice, reserving the cooking water.

⟩⟩⟩ Stir the bouillon powder into the soup along with the cavolo nero, tomatoes and butter and cook for another 3 minutes, part-covered. Stir in half the remaining herbs, the cooked rice and about 200ml/7fl oz/scant 1 cup of the reserved cooking water to thin the soup, if needed. Stir until combined and season with salt and pepper. Serve sprinkled with the remaining herbs with lemon wedges for squeezing over and crusty bread by the side.

PART-TIME VARIATION
⟩⟩⟩ Lamb harira

This lamb alternative takes longer to cook than the vegetarian version, but the slow-cooking adds to the flavour. First, brown **700g/1lb 9oz cubed lamb shoulder** in **2 tbsp olive oil**. (You will have to do this in two batches). Return the lamb to the pan when browned and add the onions and the rest of the ingredients, omitting the chickpeas and half the cavolo nero, then cook the soup for 1–1½ hours until the lamb is tender. Meanwhile, cook the rice and continue the recipe as described above.

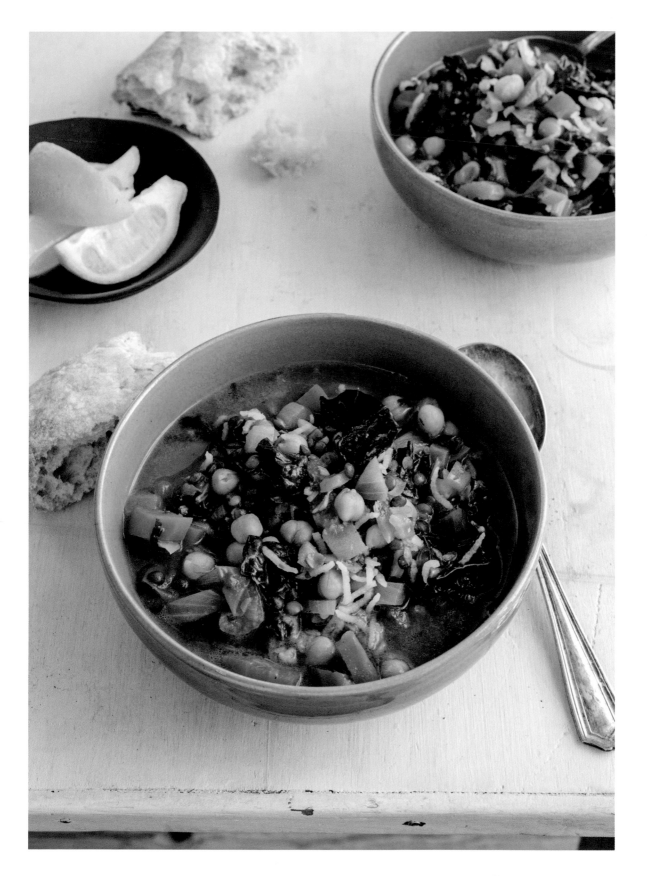

Puy lentil cassoulet
WITH walnut crust

SERVE 4–6

Preparation time ⟩ 20 minutes
Cooking time ⟩ 55 minutes

2 tbsp olive oil
1 large onion, sliced
1 leek, halved lengthways and sliced
4 garlic cloves, peeled and left whole
2 large carrots, halved lengthways and
    cut into bite-size chunks
2 turnips, peeled and cut into bite-size
    chunks
1 celery stalk, sliced
750ml/26fl oz/3¼ cups vegetable stock
2 tsp dried thyme
1 bay leaf
10cm/4in sprig of rosemary
2 tbsp tomato purée/paste
100g/3½oz/½ cup dried Puy lentils
400g/14oz can haricot beans, drained
sea salt and freshly ground black
    pepper

⟩⟩⟩ Walnut crust
70g/2½oz/¾ cup walnut pieces
2 tbsp olive oil
100g/3½oz/1⅔ cups day-old fresh
    breadcrumbs
1 garlic clove, finely chopped

Warming and comforting, this rustic, peasant-style cassoulet is loosely based on the French meaty equivalent (see opposite page), yet it works brilliantly with the earthiness of the Puy lentils and lots of veg. The crust of garlicky walnut crumbs also adds that extra something. Serve in large shallow bowls with crusty bread for dunking and a crisp green salad.

⟩⟩⟩ Heat the oil in a large heavy-based casserole over a medium heat. Add the onion and cook for 5 minutes until softened then stir in the leek, garlic, carrots, turnips and celery and sauté for another 5 minutes.

⟩⟩⟩ Pour in the stock and add the herbs, tomato purée/paste, lentils and beans. Bring to the boil, stir well, then turn the heat down and simmer for 45 minutes, covered, until the lentils are tender (remove the rosemary after 20 minutes). Stir the cassoulet occasionally to prevent it sticking and only part-cover the pan if you find you need to cook off some of the liquid. Season with salt and pepper to taste.

⟩⟩⟩ Meanwhile, make the walnut crust. Put the walnuts in a large dry frying pan and toast over a medium heat for 5 minutes, tossing regularly, until starting to colour. Remove from the pan and roughly chop. Pour the oil into the pan, add the breadcrumbs and toast, stirring regularly so that they cook evenly, for 5 minutes until turning golden. Stir in the garlic and walnuts and cook for another minute.

⟩⟩⟩ Stir a third of the walnut crust mixture into the cassoulet, then serve in large bowls, sprinkled with the remaining crust mixture.

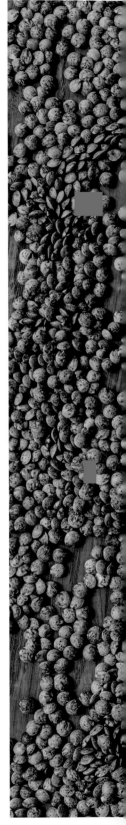

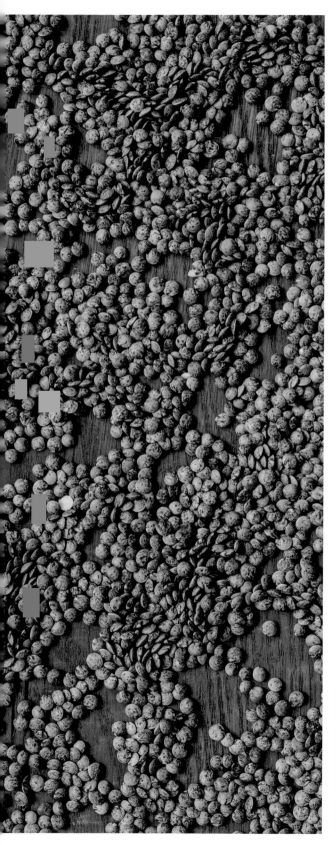

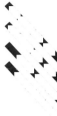

PART-TIME VARIATION
››› Pork and bean cassoulet

In keeping with the French classic, this cassoulet includes cheap cuts of meat, but not in the volume that is traditional.

Preheat the oven to 150°C/300°F/Gas 2. Brown **550g/1lb 4oz pork belly slices** and **4 Toulouse sausages** in **2 tbsp olive oil** in a flameproof casserole in batches until golden all over. This will take about 5 minutes per batch. Cut the pork and sausages into large pieces and leave to one side while you sauté the vegetables as described previously (omitting the leek and turnip).

Return the meat to the pan with the stock and remaining ingredients (omitting the lentils) and bring to the boil. Cover with the lid and cook in the oven for 1½ hours until the meat is tender and the stock has reduced. (Remove the lid for the last 30 minutes to thicken the sauce.) Meanwhile, prepare the garlicky breadcrumbs as described (omitting the walnuts) and stir half into the cassoulet just before serving. Serve sprinkled with the remaining breadcrumbs and **1 handful of chopped parsley leaves**.

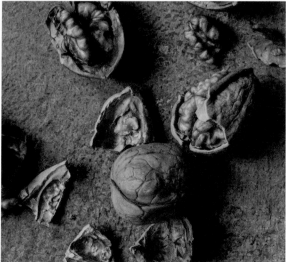

PICKLES & FERMENTS

Traditionally a way of preserving vegetables to extend their shelf life as well as add flavour before the days of refrigeration, most cultures have their own version of pickled and fermented foods. What's most interesting is that they are currently experiencing a revival in popularity, partly due to a renaissance in the back-to-basics approach in the kitchen but also because of their numerous health benefits, particularly supporting the immune system and aiding digestion.

Fermented foods such as the Wild Sauerkraut, below, are made by adding salt to vegetables to stop them going off, while leaving them at room temperature to allow the natural bacteria and wild yeasts found in the environment and the cabbage leaves to preserve them. This results in the vegetables developing a softer texture and a mildly acidic flavour. Pickles on the other hand rely on a combination of salt and vinegar as a preservative and tend to have a more piquant flavour.

The technique for making both pickles and ferments is quite straightforward, but the end result requires a certain amount of patience as it can take weeks before they are ready to eat. Bearing this in mind, here are a few speedy 'cheats' versions, when time won't wait.

⟩⟩⟩ Wild sauerkraut

This basic recipe for sauerkraut can easily be adapted with the addition of spices, such as fennel seeds, caraway seeds, chilli and ginger, or by adding other vegetables, including kohlrabi, radish or kale. Put 750g/1lb 10oz shredded green cabbage, 2 grated carrots and 2 grated turnips in a large mixing bowl. Stir in 4 tsp fine sea salt with 5 crushed peppercorns and 2 tsp crushed coriander seeds. With clean hands, turn and lightly squeeze the vegetables for 5 minutes until they start to soften and release their liquid. Leave to stand for 10 minutes.

Spoon into a sterilized glass mason or kilner jar, pressing the vegetables down firmly with the end of a rolling pin as you go to make sure they are tightly packed and until the level of the squeezed liquid is above the vegetables. Put a glass or smaller jar, inside the mason jar and weight it down to keep the vegetables submerged. Cover with a clean dish towel and secure with a rubber band to let the sauerkraut breathe. Leave at room temperature for 5–14 days, checking daily to make sure the vegetables are submerged, pushing them down if needed and removing any scum that forms on the top. Taste and when happy with the flavour, secure the lid and transfer to the refrigerator. It will keep for up to 6 months chilled.

⟫⟫ Easy kimchi

For a speedy version of kimchi, the famous and increasingly popular Korean fermented pickle, mix together a **thinly sliced 2.5cm/1in piece of fresh root ginger, 1 shredded carrot, 1 handful of shredded Chinese leaves, 2 shredded spring onions/scallions, 1 diced red chilli** and **2 tbsp toasted sesame seeds** (see method on page 98) with **4 tbsp rice vinegar, 4 tsp caster/granulated sugar** and **½ tsp salt**. Stir well and leave at room temperature for 30 minutes to allow the flavours to combine and develop. Transfer to a bowl to serve straightaway or to an airtight container and store in the refrigerator for up to 1 week.

⟫⟫ Pickled ginger

Liven up sushi, rice and noodle dishes with this simple recipe for pickled ginger, which, unlike most shop-bought alternatives, is natural coloured, rather than artificial pink. Mix together **4 tbsp rice vinegar** and **2 tbsp caster/granulated sugar** in a shallow bowl until the sugar dissolves. Add a **5cm/2in piece of fresh root ginger**, peeled and cut into paper-thin slices, and turn until coated. Leave the ginger for about 30 minutes to steep, or until softened. The ginger is ready to eat but can be kept in an airtight container in the refrigerator for up to 2 weeks.

⟫⟫ Cheat's preserved lemons

Usually preserved lemons can take weeks to ferment, but this quick and easy version makes a surprisingly good alternative to the real thing. Simply, pare the zest of **2 large lemons** into strips using a vegetable peeler and put them in a small pan. Squeeze in the **juice of 2 large lemons** and stir in **½ tsp sea salt**. Set the pan over a low heat and simmer for 8–10 minutes, or until the skin is very tender and has darkened slightly in colour. Transfer to a bowl to serve straightaway or spoon into an airtight container and store in the refrigerator for up to 1 week.

Crumbed goats' cheese ON pea purée

SERVES >>> **4**

Preparation time > 20 minutes

Cooking time > 11 minutes

115g/4oz/scant 1 cup plain/
   all-purpose flour

2 large eggs

115g/4oz/scant 2 cups day-old
   fresh breadcrumbs

finely grated zest of 1 lemon

400g/14oz rindless goats' cheese log,
   sliced into 12 x 1cm/½in thick
   rounds

olive oil, for frying

2 leeks, thinly sliced diagonally

2 handfuls of watercress or pea
   shoots (optional)

sea salt and freshly ground black
   pepper

crusty bread, to serve

>>> Pea purée

500g/1lb 2oz/4 cups frozen peas

5 tbsp double/heavy cream

80ml/2½fl oz/⅓ cup hot vegetable
   stock

There's something comforting about vegetable purées – maybe it has something to do with their similarity to baby food. Cauliflower, celeriac, parsnip, sweet potato, leek, peas and Jerusalem artichokes are all delicious blended until smooth and creamy, and when flavoured with garlic, herbs, spices and/or a dairy element you can add a new lease of life to the most everyday vegetables.

>>> Put the flour on a plate and season with a little salt and pepper. Beat the eggs in a shallow bowl and combine the breadcrumbs and lemon zest on a separate plate. Dust both sides of each slice of goats' cheese in the flour, then dunk it into the egg and finally dip into the lemony crumbs until evenly coated. Repeat until all 12 rounds of cheese are coated in the crumbs.

>>> Heat enough oil to generously cover the base of a large non-stick frying pan and fry the cheese in two batches for 2 minutes on each side until crisp and light golden. Drain on paper towels and keep warm in a low oven while you cook the second batch. Meanwhile, steam the leeks for 3 minutes until tender.

>>> To make the pea purée, cook the peas in boiling water for 3 minutes, or until tender. Drain the peas and return them to the pan with the cream and hot stock, then blend to a purée using a stick/immersion blender. Season with salt and pepper to taste and reheat, if needed.

>>> Spoon the purée onto serving plates, then top with the leeks and the crumbed goats' cheese and watercress, if using. Serve with crusty bread.

PART-TIME VARIATION
>>> Crumbed salmon on pea purée

For non-vegetarians, try topping the pea purée with a salmon fillet – incidentally both make a great dinner party dish. Preheat the oven to 200°C/400°F/Gas 6. Mix together **55g/2oz/scant 1 cup day-old fresh breadcrumbs** with the **finely grated zest of 1 lemon, 25g/1oz/⅓ cup finely grated Parmesan** and **3 tbsp finely chopped parsley leaves** and season with salt and freshly ground black pepper. Divide the crumb mixture among **4 x 150g/5½oz salmon fillets**, sprinkling it over the top of each one and pressing down slightly.

Roast the salmon on a baking sheet for 15–20 minutes until the crust is crisp and starting to colour and the fish is just cooked. Serve with the leeks and pea purée, as described above.

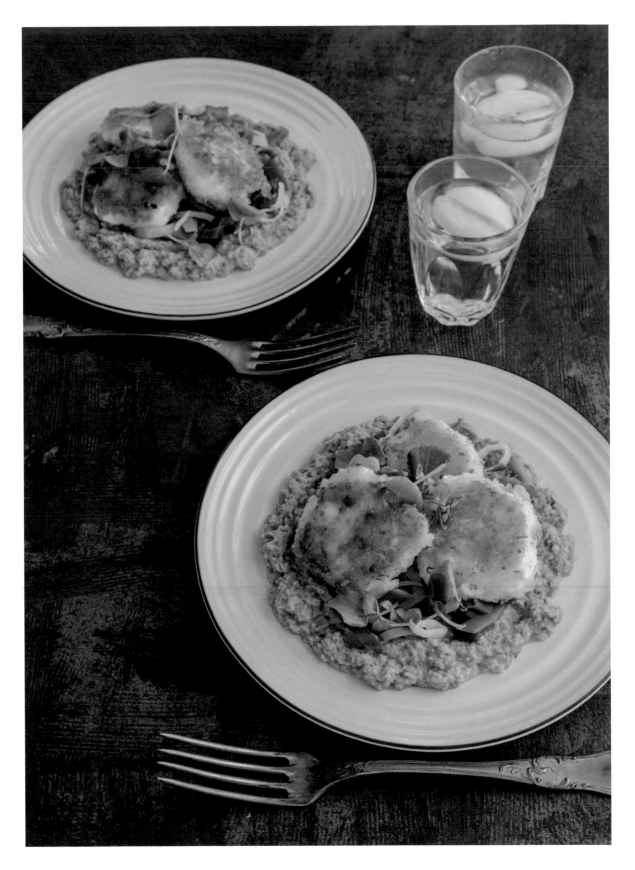

Mushroom AND Brie pancakes
WITH cider sauce

SERVES ⟩⟩⟩ **4**

Preparation time ⟩ 20 minutes, plus resting

Cooking time ⟩ 35 minutes

⟩⟩⟩ Pancakes

125g/4½oz/1 cup plain/
   all-purpose flour
large pinch of salt
1 egg, plus 1 egg yolk
300ml/10½fl oz/generous
   1¼ cups milk
sunflower oil, for frying

⟩⟩⟩ Mushroom filling

40g/1½oz/2½ tbsp butter
3 leeks, thinly sliced
300g/10½oz chestnut/cremini
   mushrooms, sliced
100g/3½oz Savoy cabbage, tough
   stalks discarded, leaves shredded
2 garlic cloves, finely chopped
1 tsp caraway seeds
100g/3½oz just-ripe Brie, rind
   removed and cut into pieces

⟩⟩⟩ Cider sauce

170ml/5½fl oz/scant ¾ cup dry cider
250ml/9fl oz/generous 1 cup
   vegetable stock
1 tbsp cornflour/cornstarch
2 tbsp milk
4 heaped tbsp crème fraîche
1 large handful of snipped chives
sea salt and freshly ground black
   pepper

For successful pancakes you need a good heavy-based, non-stick pan (preferably a shallow-sided pancake pan) and the batter needs time to rest, which allows the gluten in the flour to develop and ensures a light end result. These pancakes – slightly richer than normal thanks to the addition of an extra egg yolk – come with a creamy mushroom, Brie and Savoy cabbage filling, although they work equally well with the Chicken and Leek filling on the next page, or for sheer pancake gluttony why not serve any surplus pancakes with a sweet fruit filling.

⟩⟩⟩ First make the pancakes. Mix together the flour and salt in a large mixing bowl and make a well in the middle. Whisk together the whole egg, egg yolk and milk until combined, then pour it into the well in the bowl. Gradually draw the flour into the egg mixture, whisking to make a smooth, light batter. Leave to rest for 30 minutes.

⟩⟩⟩ While the batter is resting, make the cider sauce. Pour the cider and stock into a pan and bring to the boil, then leave to gently bubble away for 10 minutes until reduced by one-third and there is no aroma of alcohol. Mix the cornflour/cornstarch into the milk, turn the sauce down to a simmer and whisk in the milk mixture. Cook for 5 minutes, stirring, until smooth and thick. Add the crème fraîche and season with salt and pepper, then leave to one side.

⟩⟩⟩ To make the filling, melt the butter in a large sauté pan and fry the leeks for 3 minutes, then add the mushrooms, cabbage, garlic and caraway seeds and cook for another 3 minutes, stirring occasionally. Season with salt and pepper to taste, then leave to one side.

⟩⟩⟩ To make the pancakes, heat a heavy-based, non-stick frying pan over a medium heat. Pour in a little oil and wipe it over the base using a scrunched up piece of paper towel. Pour in enough batter to thinly coat the base of the pan and cook for 1 minute, flip the pancake over and cook for another 30 seconds, or until ready. Remove from the pan and keep warm in a low oven while you make seven more pancakes.

⟩⟩⟩ When the pancakes are almost ready, reheat the mushroom filling and stir in the Brie until just melted. Add the chives to the sauce and reheat briefly so the herbs keep their colour. Serve two pancakes per person, filled with the mushroom mixture and topped with the cider sauce.

PART-TIME VARIATION
»»» Chicken and leek pancakes

This chicken and leek filling is an alternative to the mushroom and Brie, opposite, but the recipes for the pancakes and the cider sauce remain the same for both dishes. As the pancakes are filled just before serving, this means it's possible to serve both fillings at the same time and appease all eating preferences in one go.

To make the filling, slice **450g/1lb skinless, boneless chicken breasts** into strips and omit the mushrooms. Heat **20g/¾oz/1½ tbsp butter** and **1 tbsp olive oil** in a large sauté pan over a medium heat. Add the chicken and fry for 5 minutes until browned all over. Remove the chicken from the pan with a slotted spoon and add **3 thinly sliced leeks**, adding more oil, if needed, then cook for 3 minutes until softened.

Add **100g/3½oz shredded Savoy cabbage leaves**, **2 finely chopped garlic cloves** and **1 tsp caraway seeds** and cook for 3 minutes, stirring often until the cabbage wilts. Return the chicken to the pan and cook for another 2 minutes until cooked through. Season with salt and pepper to taste, then add **4 tbsp crème fraîche**, instead of the Brie, and stir until combined. Leave to one side.

Cook the pancakes as described on the previous page.

Gently reheat the chicken and leek filling, adding **1 large handful of snipped chives**. Serve two pancakes per person, filled with the chicken and leek mixture and topped with the cider sauce.

Smoked cheese potato cakes <u>WITH</u> crispy kale

SERVES ⟩⟩⟩ 4

Preparation time ⟩ 20 minutes

Cooking time ⟩ 50 minutes

750g/1lb 10oz white potatoes, peeled and quartered

1½ tbsp butter

4 handfuls of cherry tomatoes

olive oil, for frying, plus extra for brushing and drizzling

4 large handfuls of curly kale, tough stalks discarded, torn into large bite-size pieces

3 smoked garlic cloves or regular garlic

100g/3½oz/heaped 1 cup grated smoked Cheddar cheese

2 hard-boiled eggs, peeled and grated

4 tbsp capers, rinsed, patted dry and roughly chopped

1 large handful of chopped flat-leaf parsley leaves

flour, for dusting

sea salt and freshly ground black pepper

⟩⟩⟩ Caper mayonnaise

6 tbsp mayonnaise

juice of ½ lemon

1 tbsp drained capers, rinsed, patted dry and finely chopped

1 tbsp nori flakes or 2 tbsp finely chopped flat-leaf parsley leaves

If possible, use a naturally smoked Cheddar in the potato cakes, rather than a smoke-flavoured one, which can lack the intensity of flavour and requisite dry texture. The smoked garlic embellishes the overall smokiness of the potato cakes, but you could use regular garlic instead.

⟩⟩⟩ Preheat the oven to 190°C/375°F/Gas 5. Cook the potatoes in plenty of boiling salted water for 12–15 minutes, or until tender. Drain and return the potatoes to the hot pan to dry briefly. Leave until cool enough to handle (or use rubber gloves) and coarsely grate into a large mixing bowl. Mix in the butter.

⟩⟩⟩ While the potatoes are cooking, brush the tomatoes with oil, place in a roasting pan, season with salt and pepper, and roast for 20 minutes, or until softened and starting to blacken, then leave to one side. Reduce the oven to 150°C/300°F/Gas 2. Toss the kale in a little oil, season with salt and pepper, and place in the roasting pan in an even layer. Roast the kale for 10–15 minutes, turning once, until crisp. Keep an eye on it as it can easily burn.

⟩⟩⟩ Meanwhile, blanch the smoked garlic in a small pan of simmering water for 2 minutes until softened. Drain and roughly chop, then gently fold into the potatoes with the Cheddar, eggs, capers and parsley and season with salt and pepper to taste.

⟩⟩⟩ Cover a plate with flour and form the potato mixture into 8 thick cakes, about 8cm/3¼in in diameter. Lightly dust each potato cake in flour. Heat enough oil to generously cover the base of a large non-stick frying pan and fry the potato cakes in two batches for 3 minutes on each side until crisp and golden. Drain on paper towels and keep warm in the bottom of the oven with the tomatoes.

⟩⟩⟩ While the potato cakes are cooking, mix together all the ingredients for the caper mayonnaise. Serve the potato cakes with the roasted tomatoes and crispy kale and with the caper mayo by the side.

PART-TIME VARIATION

⟩⟩⟩ Salmon potato cakes

Cook the potatoes, tomatoes and kale as described above. Replace the smoked cheese, smoked garlic and hard-boiled eggs with **635g/1lb 6½oz canned salmon**, drained, skin and bones removed and fish flaked. Stir the salmon into the grated potato with **4 tbsp capers** and **1 large handful chopped flat-leaf parsley leaves**, as instructed above. Form and cook the potato cakes as described above.

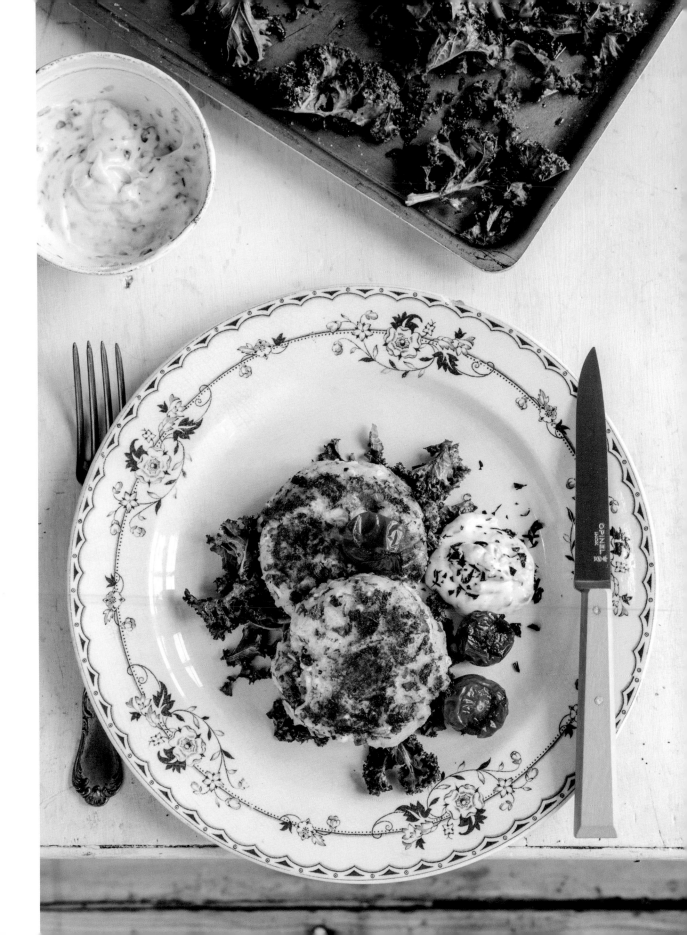

Lebanese lentils
<u>WITH</u> labneh balls

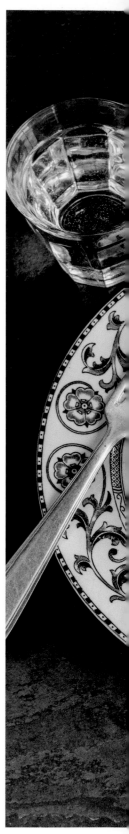

SERVES ⟩⟩⟩ 4

Preparation time ⟩ 25 minutes
Cooking time ⟩ 45 minutes

3 tbsp olive oil
1 large onion, chopped
1 heaped tbsp coriander seeds,
    crushed
1 large red pepper, deseeded
    and cut into bite-size chunks
4 carrots, halved lengthways and sliced
4 garlic cloves, chopped
200g/7oz/1¼ cups green lentils
2 tbsp tomato purée/paste
½ tsp light soft brown sugar
½ cinnamon stick
2 tsp vegetable bouillon powder
1 long red chilli, deseeded and sliced
juice of ½ large lemon
3 handfuls of chopped coriander/
    cilantro leaves
sea salt and freshly ground black
    pepper
rocket/arugula salad and flatbreads,
    warmed, to serve

⟩⟩⟩ Labneh balls
½ recipe quantity Labneh
    (see page 74)
3 tbsp sumac or chopped thyme,
    preferably lemon (optional)

The fresh yogurt cheese, labneh, is surprisingly easy to make and has a mild, slightly sour taste, which is the perfect foil to spicy food, such as this green lentil dish. A soft, crumbly goats' cheese, feta or dollops of soft cheese would make good alternatives, too, as would the Spiced Lamb Meatballs on the opposite page if you are looking for a dish to appeal to both vegetarians and meat eaters.

⟩⟩⟩ Heat the oil in a saucepan over a medium-low heat and cook the onion for 10 minutes, part-covered, until softened. Add the coriander seeds, red pepper and carrots and cook for another 3 minutes, then stir in the garlic.

⟩⟩⟩ Add the lentils, 625ml/21½fl oz/2⅔ cups water, the tomato purée/paste, sugar and cinnamon and bring to the boil, then turn the heat down and simmer for 30 minutes, part-covered, until the lentils are tender.

⟩⟩⟩ Meanwhile, take 1 tablespoon of the labneh, roll it into a ball and dip into the sumac, if using, until lightly coated.

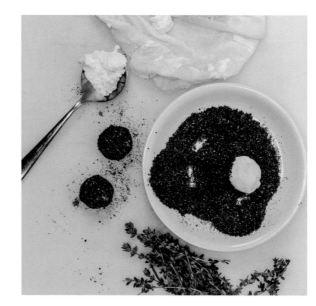

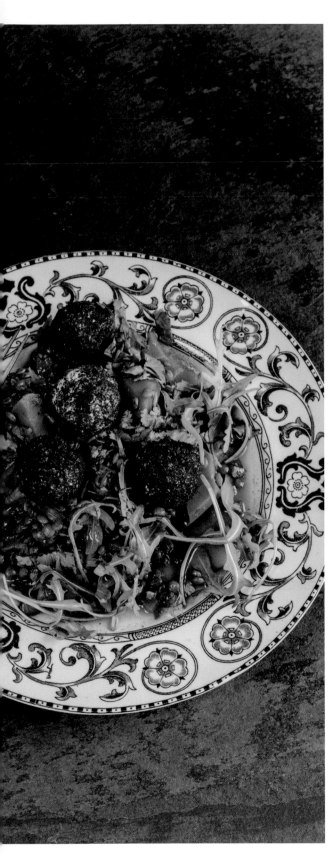

Place on a plate and repeat with the remaining labneh and sumac, then chill until ready to serve.

⟫⟫⟫ Stir the bouillon powder into the lentils with half the chilli, the lemon juice and half the coriander/cilantro, season with salt and pepper and heat through. Spoon the lentils into serving bowls, top with the labneh balls and sprinkle with the remaining coriander/cilantro and chilli. Serve with a rocket/arugula salad and warmed flatbreads.

PART-TIME VARIATION
⟫⟫⟫ Spiced lamb meatballs with lentils

Instead of the labneh balls, try these lightly spiced lamb meatballs. Toast **2 tsp cumin seeds** and **1 tbsp coriander seeds** in a large dry frying pan for 2 minutes until they smell aromatic. Grind using a pestle and mortar.

Stir **2 tbsp water** into **50g/1¾oz/scant 1 cup day-old fresh breadcrumbs**, then tip into a bowl with **400g/14oz minced/ground lamb**, the ground spices, **juice of ½ lemon**, **1 large handful of chopped mint**, **1 chopped large garlic clove** and **1 beaten egg**. Season with salt and pepper and mix together, breaking the lamb up with the back of a fork. Form into 16 walnut-size balls and chill for 30 minutes, covered, to firm up.

Heat **1 tbsp olive oil** in a large non-stick frying pan and fry the meatballs in two batches for 12 minutes, turning occasionally, until browned all over. Drain on paper towels and serve with the lentils as described above.

Tea-smoked tofu
WITH crispy ginger

SERVES ⟩⟩⟩ 4

Preparation time ⟩ 20 minutes
Cooking time ⟩ 25 minutes

800g/1lb 12oz block of tofu, drained
   well on paper towels

⟩⟩⟩ **Crispy ginger**

3 tbsp coconut or sunflower oil,
   plus extra for greasing
5cm/2in piece of fresh root ginger,
   peeled and cut into julienne strips

⟩⟩⟩ **Smoking mixture**

4 large handfuls of white rice
2 handfuls of lapsang souchong or
   black tea leaves
4 tbsp soft light brown sugar

⟩⟩⟩ **Spicy soy sauce**

4 tbsp tamari or light soy sauce
4 tbsp mirin
1 tbsp caster/granulated sugar
½ tsp shichimi togarashi or
   ¼ tsp dried chilli/hot pepper
   flakes (optional)

⟩⟩⟩ **To serve**

2 tbsp sesame seeds, toasted
   (see page 71)
2 spring onions/scallions, finely
   sliced diagonally
steamed jasmine rice

Okay, it is possible to buy ready-smoked tofu, but it's fun to have a go at smoking your own foods, and tofu is a perfect starting point as its porous texture and mild taste means it readily takes on stronger flavours. Special equipment is not needed, just a large old wok with a lid – and an open window!

⟩⟩⟩ Before you start to prepare the smoker, make the crispy ginger. Heat the oil in a large wok over a medium heat and fry the ginger for 2–3 minutes until crisp. Remove with a slotted spoon, drain on paper towels and leave to one side. Pour away the oil and wipe the wok clean.

⟩⟩⟩ Meanwhile, mix together all the ingredients for the spicy soy sauce and leave to one side.

⟩⟩⟩ To prepare the smoker, line the base and lid of the wok with foil. Put the wok on a wok stand, if you have one, to keep it stable. Put the white rice, tea and sugar in the wok and mix together. Lightly oil a wire rack and place it in the wok so it is suspended about 2cm/¾in above the smoking mixture.

⟩⟩⟩ Arrange the tofu on the rack and cover with the foil-lined lid. Heat the wok over a medium heat until you start to see little wisps of smoke escaping around the lid. Carefully patch up any leaks with foil, turn the heat to medium-low and make sure the kitchen is well ventilated. Smoke the tofu for 20 minutes, then remove the wok from the heat. When the smoke has subsided, carefully remove the lid and the rack with the tofu on it from the wok.

⟩⟩⟩ Spoon half of the sauce, half the sesame seeds and the spring onions/scallions over the steamed jasmine rice and turn until combined. Spoon the rice into serving bowls. Slice the tofu and place on top with the remaining sauce, sesame seeds and finally the crispy ginger.

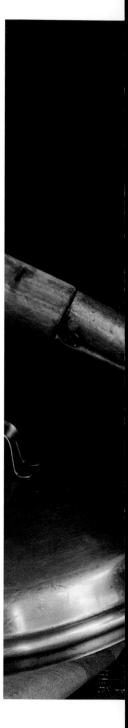

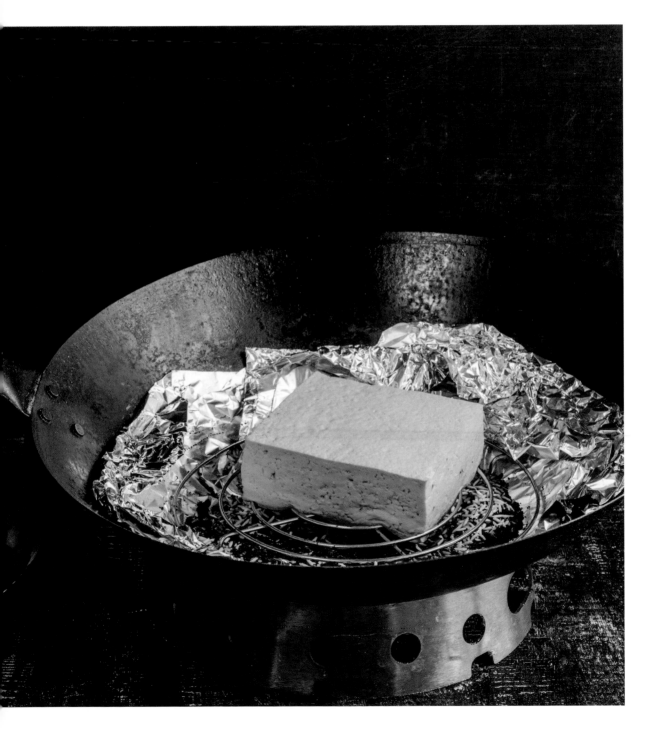

PART-TIME VARIATIONS

››› Tea-smoked chicken

Tea-smoking is a nifty cooking technique that can be adapted to all manner of different foods and it's really worth experimenting. I've had success with chicken and fish, see the recipes below, but you could also try new potatoes (par-boil them first), peppers, sweetcorn/corn cobs, garlic, salmon, prawns/shrimp and beef, just for starters.

Slice **600g/1lb 5oz skinless, boneless chicken breasts** into 2.5cm/1in wide strips. Mix together **1 tbsp olive oil** with **1 heaped tsp shichimi togarashi**, **1 tbsp light soft brown sugar** and **2 tbsp tamari** or **light soy sauce** in a large bowl. Add the chicken, turn until coated in the marinade and leave to marinate for at least 30 minutes, covered, in the refrigerator.

While the chicken is marinating, prepare the crispy ginger and spicy soy sauce as described on page 174.

To smoke the chicken, prepare the wok as instructed on the page 174. Arrange the chicken on the lightly oiled wire rack and smoke for 20 minutes following the previous instructions.

Serve the chicken with the steamed jasmine rice, spicy soy sauce and crispy ginger.

››› Tea-smoked fish

First, prepare the crispy ginger and spicy soy sauce as described on page 174.

To smoke **4 large salmon** or **trout fillets**, prepare the wok as instructed on page 174. Arrange the fish fillets, skin-side down, on the lightly oiled wire rack and smoke for 15 minutes following the previous instructions.

Serve the fish with the steamed jasmine rice, spicy soy sauce and crispy ginger.

Tempeh IN star anise broth WITH noodles

Tempeh is similar to tofu, but with a slightly nuttier, more savoury taste and firmer texture. It is equally versatile and can be roasted, fried, steamed or braised, and, like tofu, benefits from being marinated or combined with more robust flavours as here in this fragrant, gingery star anise broth.

>>> Put the cooking wine, sesame oil, soy sauce, hoisin, sugar, ginger and star anise in a deep sauté pan. Add 250ml/9fl oz/generous 1 cup water and bring to the boil, stirring until the sugar dissolves. Turn the heat down and simmer, part-covered, for 2 minutes.

>>> Add the carrots and the white part of the spring onions/scallions and simmer for 10 minutes, covered. Add the tempeh and simmer for another 10 minutes, part-covered, or until the carrots are very tender. Season and remove the star anise and ginger from the broth.

>>> Meanwhile, heat the oil in a wok or large frying pan over a high heat and stir-fry the shiitake for 5 minutes, or until starting to turn golden. At the same time, heat the noodles following the instructions on the pack, then drain. Spoon the noodles, tempeh and vegetables into large shallow bowls, pour the broth over and top with the shiitake and the green part of the spring onions/scallions.

PART-TIME VARIATION
>>> Duck with star anise broth and noodles

Replace the tempeh and shiitake with **4 duck breasts**. Preheat the oven to 200°C/400°F/Gas 6. At the same time, preheat a large dry frying pan over a medium-high heat. Score the skin of each duck breast, season with salt and pepper and place skin-side down in the pan. Sear for 7 minutes until golden and crisp, turning the heat down to medium if the duck browns too quickly. Turn the duck over and cook for 1 more minute, then transfer to a roasting pan.

Finish the duck in the oven, roasting it for 8–10 minutes until cooked but still slightly pink in the middle. Remove from the oven, cover with foil and leave to rest for 5–10 minutes.

Prepare the star anise broth as described above, reducing the quantity of water to 175ml/6fl oz/¾ cup. Cook the noodles and serve topped with the vegetables and broth. Slice the duck breasts and place on top and finish with a sprinkling of the green part of the spring onions/scallions.

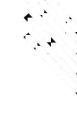

SERVES >>> **4**

Preparation time ⏺ 20 minutes
Cooking time ⏺ 25 minutes

185ml/6fl oz/¾ cup Chinese
    cooking wine or dry sherry
1 tbsp sesame oil
2 tbsp light soy sauce
4 tbsp hoisin sauce
2 tsp sugar
2.5cm/1in piece of fresh root ginger,
    peeled and sliced into rounds
2 star anise
3 carrots, sliced diagonally
3 spring onions/scallions, white and
    green parts separated, thinly sliced
    diagonally
300g/10½oz block of tempeh or tofu,
    drained well on paper towels
    and cubed
2 tbsp coconut or sunflower oil
250g/9oz shiitake mushrooms, wiped
    and stalks trimmed, halved if large
800g/1lb 12oz cooked udon noodles
sea salt and freshly ground black
    pepper

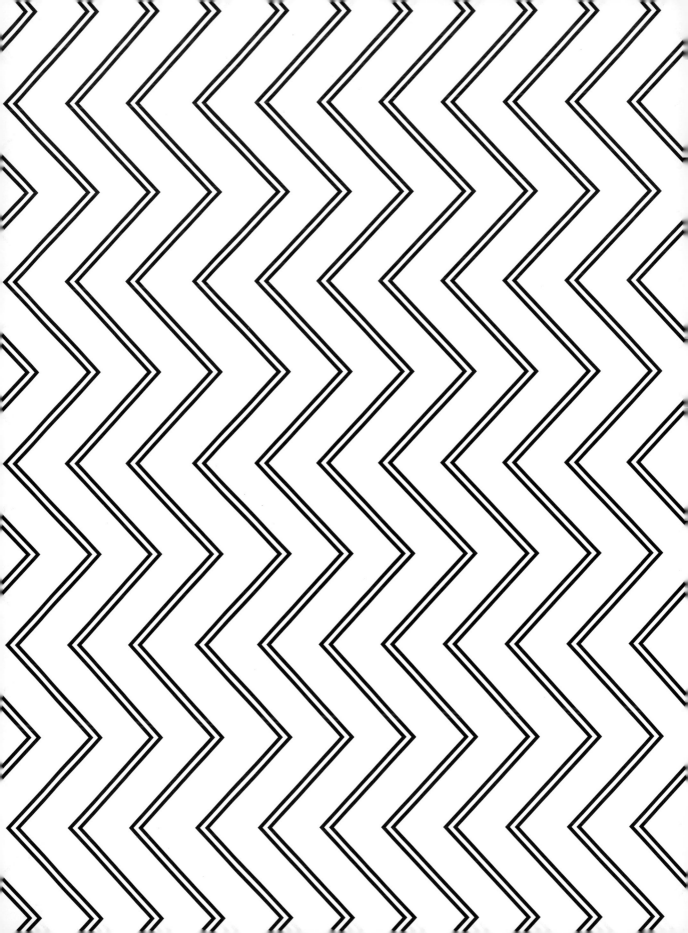

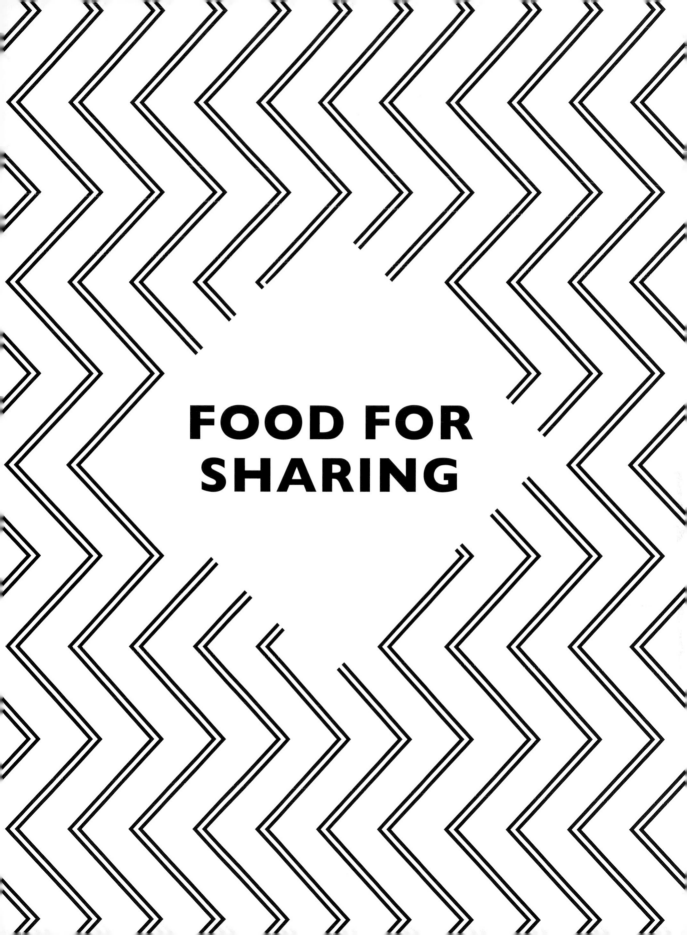

FOOD FOR SHARING

Chestnut AND porcini soup

SERVES ››› 4

Preparation time › 15 minutes,
plus soaking

Cooking time › 30 minutes

25g/1oz/1 cup dried porcini
    mushrooms
1½ tbsp butter
2 onions, chopped
1 celery stalk, thinly sliced
1 large garlic clove, chopped
2 bay leaves
1 porcini stock cube or vegetable
    stock cube
1 potato (about 300g/10½oz total
    weight), peeled and cubed
200g/7oz/1½ cups ready-cooked
    whole, peeled chestnuts, chopped
1 heaped tbsp thyme leaves, plus
    extra to serve
3 tbsp crème fraîche
40g/1½oz/⅓ cup crumbled blue
    cheese
sea salt and freshly ground black
    pepper
crusty rye bread, to serve

Originally, the full title of this recipe was 'Chestnut and porcini soup with porcini dust', but the latter sounded way too cheffy and stuffy. That said, I've struggled to come up with a better way to describe the ground dried porcini powder that is sprinkled on top of the soup before serving. This final flourish lends an intense, almost woody flavour that lifts the soup into something quite special. Likewise, porcini stock cubes are worth seeking out and can be found in some large supermarkets, Italian food stores or online. A single cube adds a deep, rich base to this soup – autumn in a bowl.

››› Put 20g/¾oz/¾ cup of the porcini in a bowl, cover with 100ml/3½fl oz/scant ½ cup just-boiled water and leave to soak for 20 minutes until softened.

››› Meanwhile, melt the butter in a large saucepan over a medium-low heat and sauté the onions for 5 minutes, part-covered and stirring regularly, until softened. Add the celery and garlic and cook for another 2 minutes.

››› Drain the porcini, reserving the soaking liquid, then finely chop. Pour the soaking liquid and 1.1 litres/38fl oz/4⅔ cups water into the onion mixture in the pan and add the bay leaves. Bring to the boil. Crumble in the stock cube and stir until dissolved, then add the soaked porcini, potato, chestnuts and thyme. Turn the heat down and simmer for 20 minutes until the vegetables are tender.

››› While the soup is cooking, put the remaining dried porcini in a grinder or use a pestle and mortar to grind them to a powder. Leave to one side.

››› Remove the bay leaves and, using a stick/immersion blender, blend the soup until smooth. Stir in the crème fraîche, season with salt and pepper, and reheat if needed. Serve in large bowls, scattered with the crumbled blue cheese, porcini powder and a few thyme leaves. Serve with slices of crusty rye bread.

Parmesan-crust fries <u>WITH</u> piri piri sauce

The Parmesan and almond crust adds a new dimension to these roasted vegetables, which make a perfect accompaniment to drinks or served as a light meal with a mixed salad, or even instead of the usual potato fries. The accompanying fresh and zingy piri piri sauce couldn't be easier to make – it's simply a blend of puréed red peppers, garlic, vinegar and paprika with no cooking required.

))) Cut each courgette/zucchini half lengthways into 6 long, thin wedges. Cut each piece of aubergine/eggplant into 8 long, thin wedges.

))) Mix together the harissa and olive oil in a large bowl, add the courgettes/zucchini, aubergine/eggplant and mushrooms and turn until the vegetables are coated in the spicy oil. Season with salt and pepper, then leave to marinate for 30 minutes, if time allows.

))) Preheat the oven to 200°C/400°F/Gas 6 and oil two large baking pans. Mix together the Parmesan and ground almonds in a shallow bowl. Dunk the vegetables, one at a time, into the Parmesan mixture until coated, then place in the prepared baking pans. Roast for 30 minutes, or until the vegetables are tender and the coating is crisp and starts to turn golden.

))) While the vegetables are roasting, make the piri piri sauce. Put the peppers, garlic, vinegar and paprika in a blender and whiz to a coarse purée. (You can also use a stick/immersion blender, blending the sauce in two batches.) Season with salt and pepper to taste. Serve the vegetables with the sauce for dipping.

SERVES))) **4**
Preparation time) 20 minutes, plus marinating
Cooking time) 30 minutes

2 courgettes/zucchini, halved crossways
1 aubergine/eggplant, cut into thirds crossways (or cut into quarters if very long)
3 tsp harissa paste
5 tbsp olive oil, plus extra for greasing
200g/7oz button mushrooms, stalks trimmed
100g/3½oz/1½ cups finely grated Parmesan cheese
80g/2¾oz/heaped ¾ cup ground almonds
sea salt and freshly ground black pepper

))) Piri piri sauce
2 large red peppers, deseeded and chopped
1 garlic clove, peeled and halved
2 tbsp red wine vinegar
1 tsp paprika

Black rice, peanut, tofu <u>AND</u> mango salad

SERVES ⟩⟩⟩ **4**

Preparation time ⟩ 20 minutes

Cooking time ⟩ 30 minutes

175g/6oz/heaped ¾ cup black rice, rinsed

55g/2oz/heaped ⅓ cup unsalted peanuts

coconut oil, or cold-pressed rapeseed/ canola oil, for frying

400g/14oz block of tofu, drained well on paper towels and cubed

1 small red onion, diced

3 spring onions/scallions, thinly sliced diagonally

1 large red chilli, deseeded and thinly sliced

85g/3oz/scant 1 cup mangetout/snow peas, thinly sliced diagonally

½ cucumber, quartered, deseeded and diced

1 large handful of chopped coriander/ cilantro leaves

1 handful of chopped mint leaves

1 large ripe mango, peeled, pitted and flesh cubed

1 recipe quantity Sesame and Lime Dressing (see page 101)

The contrast of black rice, orange mango, green herbs and red chilli makes a visually stunning dish, but the variation in textures – crisp, crunchy and soft – as well as flavours – hot, sweet and sour – also add to the overall appeal of this Asian salad. If you can't find black rice, you could use brown basmati, Camargue red rice or perhaps bulgur wheat instead – ideally you want a grain that holds its shaped when cooked.

⟩⟩⟩ Put the rice in a saucepan and cover generously with cold water. Bring to the boil, then turn the heat down to low, cover and simmer for 25–30 minutes until tender. Drain and tip the rice into a large serving bowl.

⟩⟩⟩ Meanwhile, toast the peanuts in a large dry frying pan for 5 minutes, tossing the pan occasionally until they start to colour and smell toasted. Tip onto a plate and leave to cool, then chop roughly.

⟩⟩⟩ Heat enough oil to generously cover the base of a large non-stick frying pan over a medium heat. Fry the tofu in three batches for 5 minutes, turning once, until golden and crisp, adding more oil when needed. Drain on paper towels.

⟩⟩⟩ Add the red onion, spring onions/scallions, half the chilli, the mangetout/snow peas, cucumber, half the herbs and three-quarters of the mango to the cooked rice. Pour the dressing over, then turn gently until everything is combined.

⟩⟩⟩ Spoon the dressed black rice salad onto four serving plates and top with the crisp tofu, the remaining mango, herbs and finally the peanuts.

PART-TIME VARIATION

⟩⟩⟩ Black rice, chicken and mango salad

For an alternative to the tofu, mix together **2 tsp** Thai seven-spice with **2 tbsp** cold-pressed rapeseed/canola oil or melted coconut oil in a large shallow dish, then season with salt and pepper. Slice **400g/14oz skinless, boneless chicken breasts** into strips and add to the dish. Turn the chicken in the marinade and leave to marinate for 30 minutes, if time allows.

Heat a large wok over a medium-high heat and tip in the chicken and its marinade. Stir-fry for 5–7 minutes until the chicken is cooked through and golden. Serve the chicken in place of the tofu.

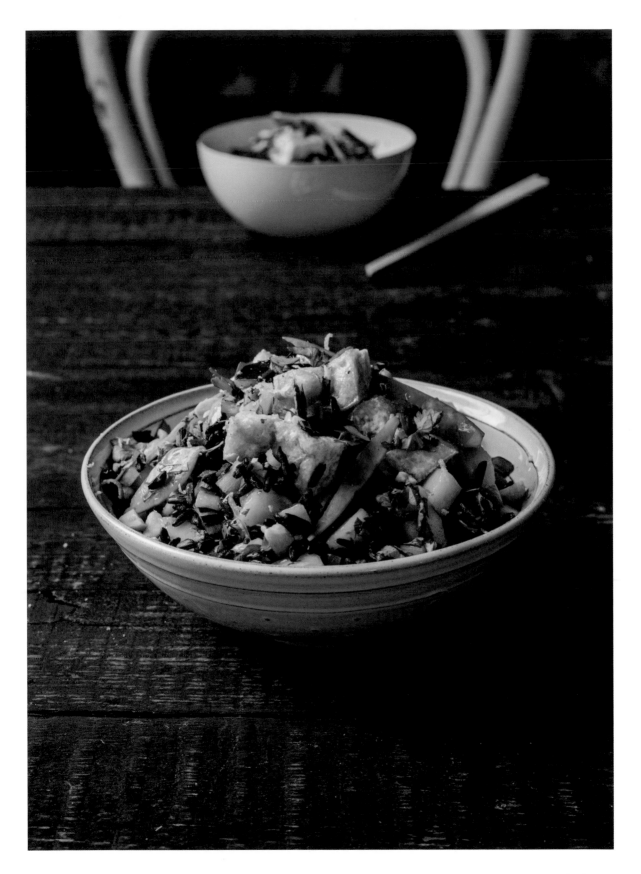

Rösti cups <u>WITH</u> beet <u>AND</u> orange relish

MAKES ››› **12**

Preparation time › 20 minutes
Cooking time › 30 minutes

400g/14oz potatoes, such as Maris
    Piper or King Edward, peeled
1 egg, lightly beaten
2 tbsp butter, melted
½ tsp sea salt
freshly ground black pepper
sprigs of dill, to serve

››› Beetroot/beet relish

250g/9oz uncooked beetroot/beets,
    peeled and cut into small dice
juice of 1 orange
finely grated zest of ½ orange
1 star anise
4 tsp balsamic vinegar
2 tsp light soft brown sugar

››› Horseradish filling

200g/7oz/1 cup crème fraîche
2 tbsp horseradish sauce
2 tsp lemon juice

A bun tray makes the perfect mould for these mini potato rösti, which are baked in the oven, rather than the more usual fried, and then filled with a horseradish cream and a star anise and orange-infused beetroot/beet relish. Alternatively, or as well as, fill the rösti cups with the salmon tartare, opposite. Both make a pretty appetizer with some salad leaves or perfect party food served with drinks.

››› Preheat the oven to 200°C/400°F/Gas 6. To make the beetroot/beet and orange relish, put all the ingredients in a saucepan with 2 tablespoons water and bring to the boil. Turn the heat down to low and simmer for 20–30 minutes, part-covered and stirring occasionally, until the beetroot/beet is tender. Check the beetroot/beet occasionally to make sure it is not drying out and add an extra splash of water, if needed. Remove the star anise and leave to cool.

››› Meanwhile, using a box grater, coarsely grate the potatoes. Pile the grated potato into the middle of a clean dish towel, draw up the sides into a bundle and squeeze to remove any water so that the potatoes are as dry as possible. Put the potatoes in a mixing bowl with the egg and season with the salt and plenty of pepper, then stir well until combined.

››› Line the bases of a 12-hole bun tray with a small round of baking paper, which will make the rösti easier to remove after cooking. Brush the base and the sides of each hole with the melted butter.

››› Divide the potato mixture among the holes of the bun tray, pressing it into the bases and up the sides to make thin, shallow cups. Bake for 20–25 minutes until the potato is cooked and golden. Leave the rösti to cool slightly, then remove from the tray and peel off the baking paper.

››› Meanwhile, mix together the crème fraîche, horseradish sauce and lemon juice. Spoon the mixture into the rösti cups, then pile the beetroot/beet relish on top. Finish each cup with a small sprig of dill and serve.

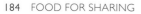

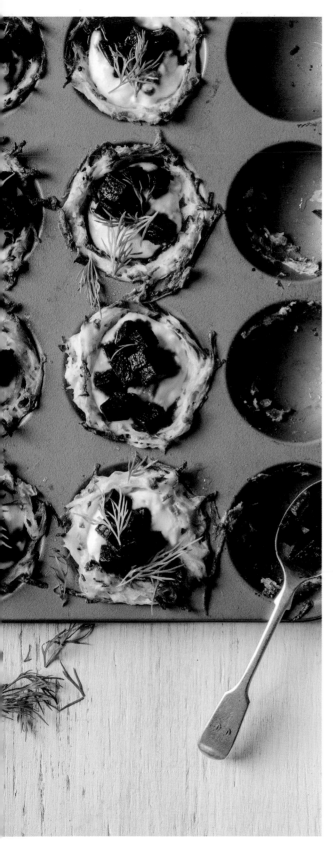

PART-TIME VARIATION

⟩⟩⟩ Rösti cups with avocado cream and salmon tartare

To make the salmon tartare, mix together 150g/5½oz very fresh diced salmon fillet, 1 finely chopped spring onion/scallion, ½ tsp finely chopped fresh root ginger, 1 large handful of chopped coriander/cilantro, 1 tsp sesame oil and the finely grated zest and juice of ½ lime.

Prepare the rösti as decribed on the previous page. Mash 2 large avocados and mix with 3 tbsp crème fraîche and the zest and juice of 1½ limes, then season with salt and pepper. Spoon the avocado mixture into the rösti cups, then top with the salmon and finely chopped red chilli.

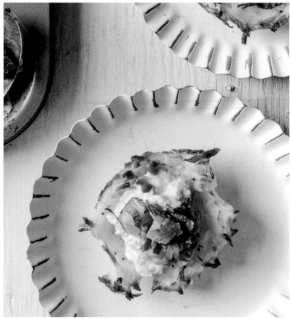

Sushi cones <u>WITH</u> pickled ginger

MAKES 20

Preparation time ⟩ 30 minutes, plus cooling

Cooking time ⟩ 15 minutes

165g/5¾oz/heaped ¾ cup sushi rice

1½ tbsp rice vinegar

2 tsp caster/granulated sugar

½ tsp salt

1 avocado, halved, pitted, peeled and cut into long, thin slices

juice of ½ lime

1 tbsp wasabi paste

5 sheets of nori, quartered

5cm/2in piece of cucumber, quartered, deseeded and cut into long, thin slices

½ small red pepper, deseeded and cut into long, thin slices

1 spring onion/scallion, trimmed and sliced diagonally into long, thin slices

20 large basil leaves

1 recipe quantity Pickled Ginger (see page 165) and tamari or light soy sauce, to serve

Surprisingly easy to make, these sushi cones don't require any specialist rolling mats or any other kitchen gadgetry… simply gather a few friends together around the dining table, then make and eat as you go. You could serve a combination of the vegetable and smoked trout fillings, to cater for all food tastes.

⟩⟩⟩ First prepare the sushi rice. Rinse the rice three times and drain well, then transfer to a saucepan. Pour 350ml/12fl oz/scant 1½ cups water into the pan, give it a quick stir, then bring to the boil. Turn the heat down to low and simmer for 12–15 minutes, covered, until tender and the water has been absorbed. Remove the pan from the heat and leave to stand for 5 minutes, covered.

⟩⟩⟩ Meanwhile, mix together the rice vinegar, sugar and salt. Transfer the rice to a shallow dish, gently stir in the rice vinegar mixture using a wooden spoon, then leave to cool.

⟩⟩⟩ Turn the avocado in the lime juice until coated to prevent it discolouring.

⟩⟩⟩ To make the rolls, smear a dot of wasabi over each square of nori. Place 2–3 teaspoons of the cooled rice diagonally across the middle of each square, then top with a slice of avocado, a slice or two of cucumber, red pepper and spring onion/scallion. Top with a basil leaf. Wet the edge of the nori and roll into a cone shape, pressing the edge to seal. Repeat to make 20 cones in total and serve with small bowls of pickled ginger and tamari for dipping.

PART-TIME VARIATION
⟩⟩⟩ Smoked trout and avocado sushi cones

Slice 125g/4½oz smoked trout into 20 long strips and use as a filling for the sushi cones with the rice, avocado and cucumber, in place of the red pepper and spring onion/scallion. You could also try slices of hot-smoked trout, smoked mackerel or cooked prawns/shrimp.

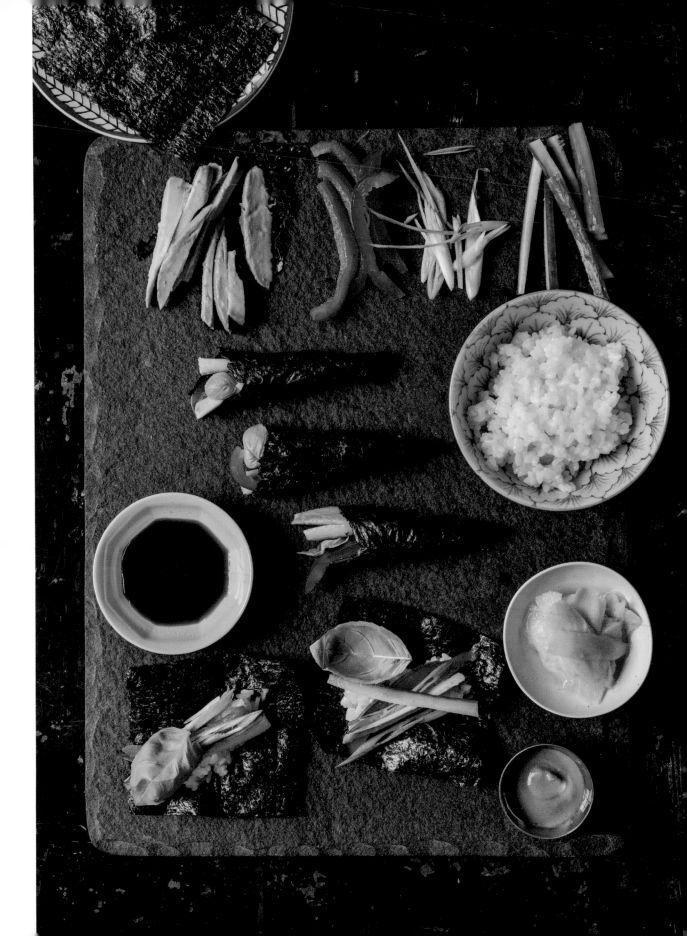

Dosa <u>WITH</u> coconut <u>AND</u> lime chutney

SERVES ›› **4**

Preparation time › 20 minutes, plus resting

Cooking time › 50 minutes

100g/3½oz/½ cup basmati rice, rinsed
½ tsp instant dried yeast
135g/4¾oz/¾ cup rice flour
½ tsp sea salt
1 tsp nigella seeds
1 tsp turmeric
100g/3½oz/generous ⅓ cup plain yogurt
a squeeze of lime juice
cold-pressed rapeseed/canola oil, for frying

›› Coconut and lime chutney

75g/2½oz/1 cup unsweetened desiccated/dried shredded coconut
juice of 1 large lime
1 tsp finely grated lime zest
2 handfuls of finely chopped coriander/cilantro leaves
2 handfuls of finely chopped mint leaves
2 green chillies, deseeded and finely chopped
sea salt

Traditionally, the batter for an Indian dosa takes days to ferment, but the batter for these light rice flour pancakes makes a comparatively quick alternative and without compromising on flavour. Delicious eaten as a prequel to the koftas (see opposite) with generous spoonfuls of the fresh coconut chutney, the dosa can also be served as an accompaniment to curries and other spicy dishes or as a wrap for the Saag Aloo (see page 86).

›› Put the rice in a saucepan and pour in enough water to cover by about 1cm/½in. Bring to the boil, then turn the heat down to its lowest setting, cover, and simmer for 10 minutes, or until tender and the water has been absorbed. Remove the pan from the heat and leave to rest for 5 minutes.

›› Meanwhile, stir the yeast into 3 tablespoons lukewarm water. Leave for 5 minutes until it starts to froth.

›› Mix together the flour, salt, nigella seeds and turmeric in a large mixing bowl.

›› Transfer the cooked rice to a blender with the yogurt, lime juice and 650ml/22½fl oz/2¾ cups lukewarm water and blend to a smooth paste. Spoon into the bowl containing the flour mixture and stir in the yeast to make a batter. Cover with cling film/plastic wrap and leave in a warm place for 2–3 hours until slightly risen, frothy and light.

›› While the batter is resting, make the coconut and lime chutney. Put the coconut in a bowl and stir in the lime juice and 185ml/6fl oz/¾ cup water and leave to one side for 10 minutes. Stir in the lime zest, herbs and chillies and season with salt. Leave at room temperature until ready to serve.

›› To make the dosa, heat a large dry frying pan over a medium heat and brush the surface with a little oil. Add 100ml/3½fl oz/scant ½ cup of the batter in an even layer (it is easiest to start pouring it from the middle and work your way out) and cook for 4–5 minutes, turning once, to make a thin, golden, slightly crisp pancake. Keep the dosa warm in a low oven while you make eight in total, allowing for a few mishaps. Serve warm with the chutney.

Paneer koftas IN spiced yogurt sauce

Paneer, the Indian fresh mild cheese, has a dense, slightly crumbly texture and makes the perfect neutral base for these lightly spiced, crisp balls. You can find it sold in blocks in the chiller cabinet of large supermarkets and Asian grocers. The koftas can be served with the dosa and chutney (see previous page) or with basmati rice, or warm naan bread.

》》》 To make the koftas, cook the potatoes in plenty of boiling salted water for 12–15 minutes until tender.

》》》 Meanwhile, to make the spiced yogurt sauce, toast the cardamom and coriander seeds in a large dry frying pan over a medium-low heat for 1–2 minutes until they start to smell slightly toasted. Grind the seeds to a powder in a pestle and mortar.

》》》 Blend the onion, ginger and garlic together to make a paste. Heat the oil in a saucepan over a medium heat and cook the paste for 3 minutes, stirring. Stir in the ground spices, tomato purée/paste and pour in 455ml/16fl oz/ 2 cups water. Bring to the boil, then turn the heat down, add the turmeric, chilli and garam masala and simmer for 15 minutes, part-covered, until reduced and thickened. Add the yogurt and heat through gently, stirring. Season to taste with salt and pepper.

》》》 While the sauce is cooking, drain the potatoes and leave until cool enough to handle. Coarsely grate them into a mixing bowl and stir in the paneer, spices, green chilli and cornflour/cornstarch. Season and form into golf ball-size balls.

》》》 Heat enough oil to deep-fry the koftas in a large pan over a medium-high heat to 180°C/350°F (the temperature is correct when a cube of bread turns golden in 1 minute). Fry the koftas in batches for 5 minutes, or until golden all over. Remove from the pan with a slotted spoon and drain on paper towels. To serve, reheat the sauce, if necessary, and serve with the koftas.

SERVES 》》》 **4**
Preparation time 》 20 minutes
Cooking time 》 30 minutes

2 potatoes (about 375g/13oz total weight), peeled and halved
225g/8oz paneer cheese, patted dry and coarsely grated
½ tsp dried chilli/hot pepper flakes
1 tsp garam masala
1 green chilli, deseeded and finely chopped
1 tbsp cornflour/cornstarch
sea salt and freshly ground black pepper

》》》 Spiced yogurt sauce
seeds from 6 cardamom pods
1 tsp coriander seeds
1 onion
2.5cm/1in piece of fresh root ginger, peeled and roughly chopped
3 large garlic cloves, peeled
1 tbsp sunflower oil, plus extra for deep-frying
4 tbsp tomato purée/paste
½ tsp turmeric
½ tsp dried chilli/hot pepper flakes
1 heaped tsp garam masala
4 tbsp plain yogurt

Artichoke <u>AND</u> saffron ragoût <u>WITH</u> lemon aioli

SERVES ⟩⟩⟩ **4**

Preparation time ⟩ 15 minutes

Cooking time ⟩ 30 minutes

1 large pinch of saffron

4 tbsp extra virgin olive oil

50g/1¾oz/scant 1 cup day-old fresh
    breadcrumbs

3 shallots, sliced

3 courgettes/zucchini, halved
    lengthways and sliced into chunks

3 large garlic cloves, finely chopped

1 heaped tbsp drained capers, rinsed

½ tsp dried chilli/hot pepper flakes

400g/14oz can flageolet beans, drained

185ml/6fl oz/¾ cup dry white wine

350ml/12fl oz/scant 1½ cups vegetable
    stock

3 tbsp tomato purée/paste

200g/7oz chargrilled artichoke hearts
    in oil, drained, halved if large

2 large handfuls of baby spinach leaves,

sea salt and freshly ground black
    pepper

1 recipe quantity Lemon Aioli (see
    page 200) and crusty bread,
    to serve

For me, this dish reflects the cooking style and flavours of Provence in the south of France. The vegetables are cooked in a white wine and saffron broth until meltingly tender, then served topped with a sprinkling of crisp breadcrumbs and a spoonful of garlicky lemon aioli. Crusty bread to mop up the fragrant sauce is a must.

⟩⟩⟩ Put the saffron in a ramekin and pour over 1 tablespoon hot water. Stir and leave until needed.

⟩⟩⟩ Heat half the oil in a large non-stick frying pan over a medium heat and fry the breadcrumbs for 3–5 minutes, turning regularly, until golden and crisp, then leave to one side.

⟩⟩⟩ Heat the remaining oil in a large, heavy-based pan over a medium-low heat and sauté the shallots for 5 minutes, covered, until softened but not coloured. Add the courgettes/zucchini, garlic and capers and cook for another 3 minutes, stirring regularly, until tender, then add the red pepper flakes and beans.

⟩⟩⟩ Pour in the wine and allow to gently bubble away for 5 minutes until reduced and there is no aroma of alcohol. Add the stock and tomato purée/paste, stir well and simmer over a medium-low heat for 10 minutes, part-covered, until the liquid has reduced.

⟩⟩⟩ Stir in the artichokes and spinach, season with salt and pepper and simmer for 2 minutes until the spinach has wilted. Serve in large, shallow bowls sprinkled with the breadcrumbs and topped with a large spoonful of aioli. Serve with thick slices of crusty bread for dunking.

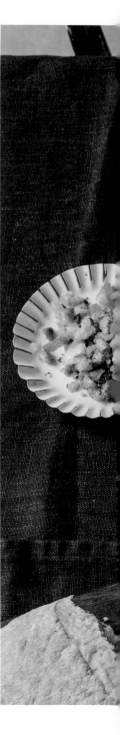

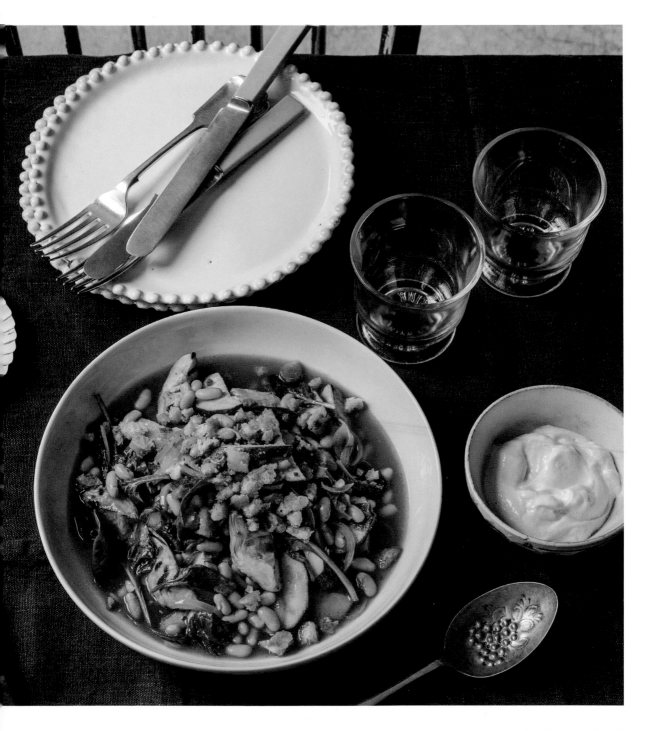

PART-TIME VARIATION

››› Provençal seafood ragoût

For a seafood twist on the vegetarian dish on the previous page, prepare the saffron and breadcrumbs following the instructions on page 190. Meanwhile, cook the shallots as described, then add **2 sliced courgettes/zucchini** and **3 chopped anchovy fillets** in place of the capers. Cook for another 3 minutes, stirring regularly, until tender, then add the red pepper flakes (omitting the beans). Continue the recipe, adding the ingredients for the sauce as described.

Replace the artichokes and spinach with **300g/10½oz thick white fish fillet**, such as gurnard, cut into large chunks, and cook for 2 minutes, then add **300g/10½oz raw, peeled king prawns/jumbo shrimp** and cook for a further 2 minutes. Gently stir in **250g/9oz prepared squid rings** and cook for another minute. Season with salt and pepper and serve in large, shallow bowls sprinkled with the breadcrumbs and topped with a large spoonful of aioli. Serve with thick slices of crusty bread.

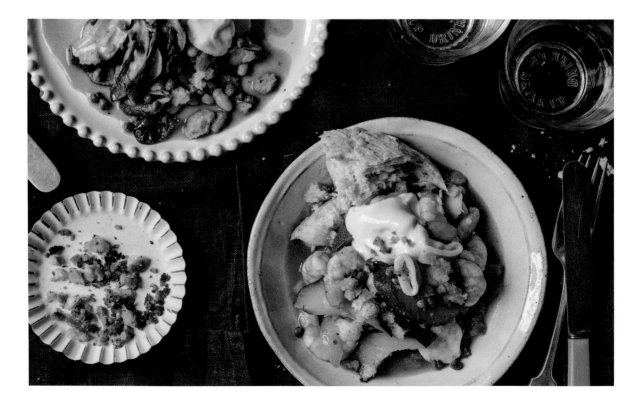

Teriyaki vegetables WITH wakame pickle

For times when you want to knock up a simple, quick, tasty meal for friends and family, this dish ticks all the right boxes. The combination of mirin, tamari, honey and ginger makes a lovely sticky-sweet glaze for the stir-fried vegetables or the mackerel, while the wakame pickle adds a tangy contrast. Look for packets of dried wakame in large supermarkets and Asian grocers. You'll find a little goes a long way as the sea vegetable swells impressively when rehydrated.

>>> To make the wakame pickle, soak it in cold water for 5 minutes until rehydrated, then drain well. Mix together the rice vinegar, mirin and sugar until the sugar dissolves, then pour it over the wakame. Stir in the shichimi togarashi and a quarter of the green parts of the spring onions/scallions, then leave to one side.

>>> To make the teriyaki sauce, put the tamari, mirin, honey and ginger in a small saucepan with 4 tablespoons water and cook over a medium heat for 2–3 minutes until reduced and thickened slightly.

>>> Meanwhile, steam the asparagus and broccoli for 2 minutes until the vegetables are slightly tender but not fully cooked. Refresh under cold running water and drain.

>>> Heat the oil in a large wok over a high heat. Add the courgettes/zucchini and edamame/soy beans and stir-fry for 2 minutes. Add the asparagus, broccoli, garlic and remaining spring onions/scallions, then stir-fry for another minute before pouring in the teriyaki sauce. Cook for a minute or so, turning constantly, until the vegetables are coated in the sauce, adding a splash more water if needed. Serve the vegetables with rice sprinkled with sesame seeds, and the wakame pickle.

PART-TIME VARIATION

>>> Teriyaki mackerel with wakame pickle

Marinate **4–8 mackerel fillets** (depending on their size) in **4 tbsp tamari** or **light soy sauce, 4 tbsp mirin, 2 tsp clear honey** and **2.5cm/1in piece of grated fresh root ginger** for at least 30 minutes. Preheat the grill/broiler to high. Remove the mackerel from the marinade and grill/broil, skin-side up, for 3 minutes, or until crisp, then turn over and grill/broil for another 2 minutes, or until cooked.

Meanwhile, pour any leftover marinade into a small pan, add 3 tbsp water and heat through. Serve the mackerel with rice and the teriyaki sauce, topped with the wakame pickle and **2 shredded spring onions/scallions.**

SERVES >>> **4**
Preparation time > 15 minutes
Cooking time > 8 minutes

400g/14oz asparagus, stalks
    trimmed
250g/9oz long-stem broccoli, trimmed
2 tbsp coconut or sunflower oil
2 courgettes/zucchini, halved
    lengthways and cut into 1cm/½in
    thick slices
125g/4½oz/1 cup edamame/soy beans
2 large garlic cloves, thinly sliced
1 tbsp sesame seeds, toasted (see
    page 71) and jasmine rice, to serve

>>> Teriyaki sauce
5 tbsp tamari or light soy sauce
4 tbsp mirin
2 tsp clear honey
2.5cm/1in piece of fresh root ginger,
    grated (no need to peel)

>>> Wakame pickle
10g/¼oz/½ cup dried wakame
    seaweed
2 tbsp rice vinegar
4 tsp mirin
1 tsp caster/granulated sugar
½–1 tsp shichimi togarashi or dried
    chilli/hot pepper flakes, to taste
4 spring onions/scallions, thinly sliced,
    white and green parts separated

Beetroot pappardelle <u>WITH</u> hazelnuts <u>AND</u> sage butter sauce

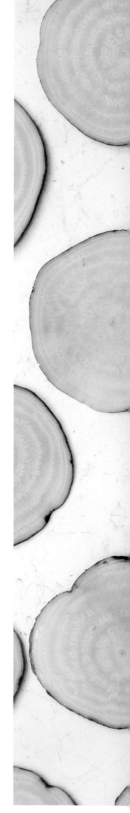

SERVES ⟩⟩⟩ **4**

Preparation time ⟩ 1¼ hours,
plus chilling

Cooking time ⟩ 55 minutes

2 onions, cut into wedges
1 whole garlic bulb
75g/2½oz/scant ½ cup shelled,
    blanched hazelnuts
250g/9oz long-stem broccoli, trimmed
100g/3½oz/7 tbsp butter
3 tbsp chopped sage
a good squeeze of lemon juice
140g/5oz rindless goats' cheese
    log, crumbled
freshly ground black pepper

⟩⟩⟩ Beetroot/beet pasta

400g/14oz raw beetroot/beets,
    trimmed, peeled and cut into
    wedges
4 tbsp olive oil
2 eggs plus 1 egg yolk
300g/10½oz/scant 2½ cups '00' flour,
    plus extra for dusting
½ tsp sea salt, plus extra to season
fine polenta/cornmeal or semolina,
    for dusting

Fresh pasta is fun to make, but admittedly it requires time and a certain amount of effort, but I'd like to think that this recipe deserves both. This makes a stunning special meal or alternative Sunday lunch, and what's more once all the preparation has been done, the fresh pasta takes next to no time to cook. You could, of course, use ready-made pappardelle to speed things up.

⟩⟩⟩ Preheat the oven to 190°/350°F/Gas 5. To start the pasta, toss the beetroot/beets in half the olive oil in a roasting pan. Roast for 45–50 minutes, turning once, until tender, then leave to cool.

⟩⟩⟩ While the beetroot/beets are roasting, toss the onion in 1 tablespoon of the oil in a separate roasting pan and roast for 45 minutes, turning once, until tender. Leave to one side.

⟩⟩⟩ Wrap the garlic in foil and roast for 30 minutes, or until the cloves are tender. At the same time, put the hazelnuts in a roasting pan and toast in the bottom of the oven for 12–15 minutes until light golden and toasted, checking regularly to make sure they don't burn. Leave to one side.

⟩⟩⟩ To make the pasta, use a stick/immersion blender or mini food processor to purée 125g/4½oz of the roasted beetroot/beets to a coarse paste, then add the whole eggs and yolk and continue blending to form a smooth purée.

⟩⟩⟩ Sift the flour and salt into a large mixing bowl and stir until combined. Make a well in the centre, add the beetroot/beet purée and mix with a fork to form a dough – this can be done in a food processor if you prefer. Tip the dough onto a well-floured work surface and knead for 10 minutes, adding more flour if the dough is very wet, until smooth and elastic. Wrap the ball of dough in cling film/plastic wrap and leave to rest for 30 minutes. (The dough will keep for up to 1 day in the refrigerator.)

⟩⟩⟩ Take a quarter of the pasta, leaving the rest covered with cling film/plastic wrap, and press it into a flat square. Dust the dough in flour and pass it through the widest

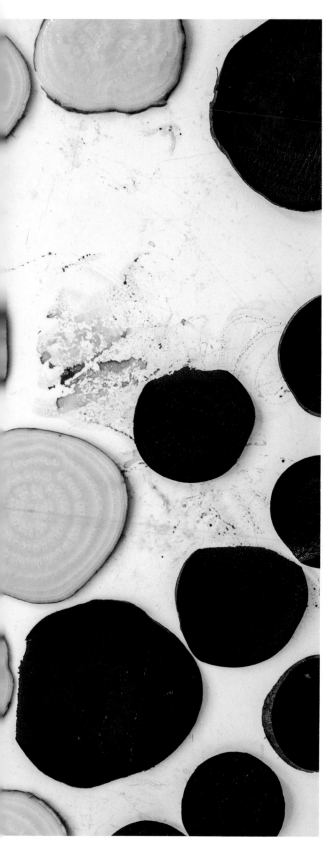

setting of a pasta machine. Fold the dough over and pass it through again, then repeat twice more. Once you have a rectangular piece of dough, turn the pasta machine down a setting and pass the dough through again. Repeat this process until you have reached the penultimate setting (the pasta has a tendency to break if taken down to the lowest setting due to the addition of beetroot/beets), lightly dusting with flour if it becomes too sticky. Cut the dough in half crossways if it becomes too long to manage. Dust a sheet of baking paper with polenta/cornmeal and put the rolled-out pasta on top to prevent it sticking. Repeat this process with the remaining dough.

⟩⟩⟩ Using a pasta cutter or sharp knife, cut the pasta into 2.5cm/1in wide strips, hanging them on the back of a chair over a dish towel or from a coat hanger to dry as you go. You can cook the pasta straight away or leave it to dry overnight, which will also help it to keep its colour during cooking.

⟩⟩⟩ Bring a large saucepan of salted water to a rolling boil. Add the broccoli and blanch for 2–3 minutes until just tender, then lift out with a slotted spoon, leaving the boiling water ready for the pasta, and refresh under cold running water.

⟩⟩⟩ Cut the remaining roasted beetroot/beets into chunks. Melt the butter and the last tablespoon of oil in a large sauté pan. Add the sage, beetroot/beets and roasted onion. Squeeze each clove of roasted garlic out of its skin into the pan, and when heated through, add the broccoli and 6 tablespoons of the broccoli cooking water. Season with pepper and add a good squeeze of lemon juice. Turn off the heat and cover the pan with a lid to keep the sauce warm.

⟩⟩⟩ Meanwhile, drop the pasta into the gently boiling water, stir, and cook for 30 seconds to 1 minute depending on how dry the pasta is – it should be just al dente when cooked. Using tongs, transfer the pasta to four large, shallow bowls and top with the buttery vegetable sauce. Scatter the hazelnuts and goats' cheese over before serving.

Red bean AND chocolate chilli

SERVES ⟩⟩⟩ **4–6**

Preparation time ⟩ 20 minutes,
plus soaking

Cooking time ⟩ 35 minutes

1 dried chipotle chilli or 1 tbsp chipotle
    paste
2 tbsp olive oil
2 onions, roughly chopped
1 celery stalk, sliced
2 carrots, quartered lengthways
    and sliced
1 tsp ground ginger
2 tsp ground cumin
½ cinnamon stick
1 tsp dried chilli/hot pepper flakes,
    or to taste
1 tsp dried oregano
2 bay leaves
180ml/6fl oz/¾ cup red wine
250ml/9fl oz/1 cup vegetable stock
400g/14oz can chopped tomatoes
2 x 400g/14oz cans red kidney beans,
    drained
10g/¼oz dark/bittersweet chocolate,
    chopped
sea salt and freshly ground black
    pepper
basmati rice and sour cream,
    to serve

The dark chocolate adds an amazing richness to this chilli, but be judicious with it as too much can soon become overpowering. A big bowl of chilli is perfect for a group gathering, especially when it's cold outside. There is also a beef version that uses the same blend of spices and flavourings. Both chillies will happily sit for a couple of days in the refrigerator if made in advance – in fact this allows time for the flavours to develop. You may wish to go easy on the chilli if serving to children.

⟩⟩⟩ Soak the dried chipotle chilli in 4 tablespoons just-boiled water for 20 minutes until softened.

⟩⟩⟩ Meanwhile, heat the oil in a large casserole over a medium-low heat and sauté the onions, covered, for 7 minutes until softened. Stir in the celery, carrots, spices and herbs and cook for another 3 minutes, stirring often.

⟩⟩⟩ Drain the chipotle, reserving the soaking water, and roughly chop, then add to the casserole with the red wine, if using. Allow to bubble away for 5 minutes until reduced and there is no aroma of alcohol.

⟩⟩⟩ Stir in the chipotle soaking water, stock, tomatoes and kidney beans. Bring to the boil, then turn the heat down and simmer for 20 minutes, part-covered, or until reduced and thickened. Season with salt and pepper to taste, and stir in the chocolate until melted into the sauce. Serve with basmati rice, topped with a spoonful of sour cream.

PART-TIME VARIATION
⟩⟩⟩ Slow-cooked beef and chocolate chilli

Heat **2 tbsp sunflower oil** in a large casserole over a medium-high heat. Add **700g/1lb 9oz brisket** or **braising steak**, cut into large chunks and cook for 5 minutes until browned all over. (You will need to do this in two batches.) Remove the beef from the casserole with a slotted spoon and continue the recipe following the instructions above up until you add the stock.

Return the beef to the pan with **250ml/9fl oz/1 cup beef stock** instead of vegetable stock and halving the quantity of kidney beans. Cook, covered, over a low heat for 1½–2 hours until the beef is tender. Part-cover the casserole towards the end of the cooking time to allow the sauce to reduce and thicken. Serve with basmati rice and a spoonful of sour cream.

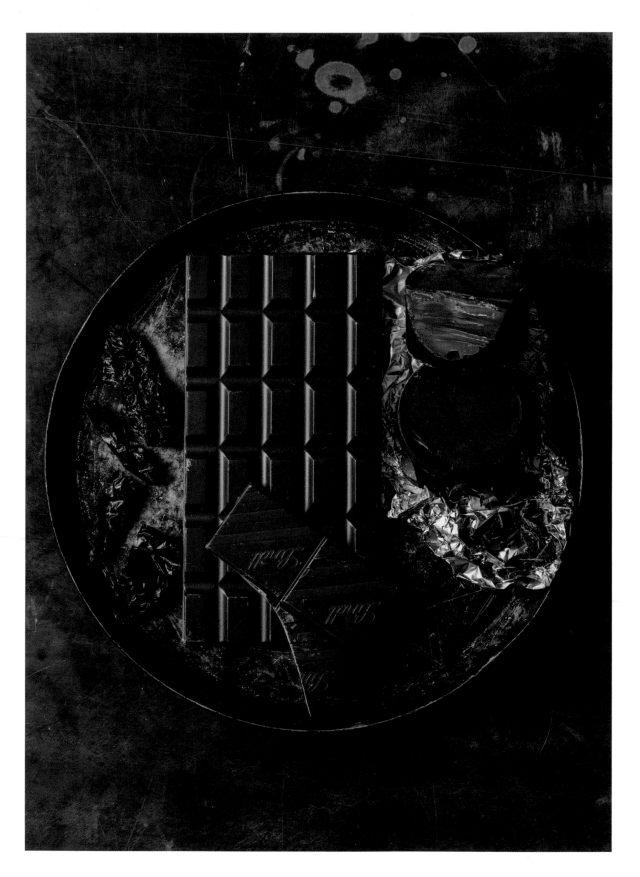

Slow-rise pan pizza

SERVES ⟩⟩⟩ **4**
Preparation time ⟩ 20 minutes,
plus overnight rise and proving
Cooking time ⟩ 40 minutes

⟩⟩⟩ **Pizza base**

4g/scant 1 tsp instant dried yeast
270–290ml/9½–10fl oz/about
    1¾ cups lukewarm water
400g/14oz/3 cups strong white flour,
    plus extra for dusting
2 tsp sea salt
3 tbsp extra virgin olive oil, plus extra
    for greasing and drizzling

⟩⟩⟩ **Tomato sauce**

1 garlic clove, finely chopped
250ml/9fl oz/generous 1 cup passata
    or sieved tomatoes
2 tsp tomato purée/paste
1 tsp dried oregano
salt and freshly ground black pepper

⟩⟩⟩ **Red onion and mushroom
    topping**

1 red onion, thinly sliced
6 chestnut/cremini mushrooms, thinly
    sliced
4 tsp drained capers
    or 1 handful of pitted black olives
250g/9oz smoked or regular
    mozzarella cheese, patted dry
    and torn into pieces
1 handful of basil leaves

This pizza takes a bit of forward planning. I find it easiest to make the dough before bedtime – it takes about 10 minutes – so it's ready to cook the following evening. The slow-rise gives the dough a wonderful depth of flavour, while the unconventional cooking method gives a surprisingly authentic crisp crust.

⟩⟩⟩ To make the dough, stir the yeast into 5 tablespoons lukewarm water and leave until it starts to froth. Meanwhile, mix together the flour and salt in a large mixing bowl and make a well in the middle. Pour in the yeasted water and 1 tablespoon of the olive oil, then gradually add about 270ml/9½fl oz/1½ cups lukewarm water, stirring initially with a fork and then with your fingers until everything comes together into a ball of dough.

⟩⟩⟩ Tip the dough onto a lightly floured work surface and knead for 10 minutes until smooth and elastic. Put the dough in the cleaned, lightly oiled bowl, cover with cling film/plastic wrap and leave overnight (it will keep until the following evening), ideally somewhere draught-free and warm, until doubled in size.

⟩⟩⟩ One hour before cooking, tip the dough out of the bowl, press down lightly and divide into four balls. Wrap each ball in a lightly oiled sheet of cling film/plastic wrap.

⟩⟩⟩ To make the sauce, heat the remaining oil and garlic in a pan over a low heat. Stir in the passata, tomato purée/paste and oregano and cook gently for 10 minutes until reduced and thickened. Seasoned with salt and pepper and leave to one side.

⟩⟩⟩ Preheat the grill/broiler to high. Roll the dough balls out, one at a time, on a lightly floured work surface into thin rounds, about 5mm/¼in thick. Heat a medium ovenproof frying pan over a medium-high heat and brush the base with oil. Carefully place the pizza base into the pan, pressing it out to the sides, and cook for 3 minutes until light golden and crisp underneath.

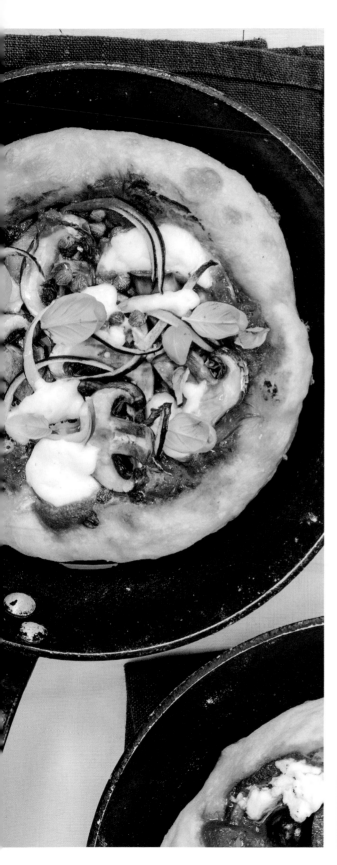

>>> Spread a few spoonfuls of the tomato sauce over the top of the pizza and scatter a quarter of the onion, mushrooms, capers and mozzarella on top. Drizzle with a little oil and grill/broil for 4 minutes until bubbling and slightly golden. Repeat with the remaining dough and toppings to make four pizzas in total. Just before serving, scatter a few basil leaves on top.

PART-TIME VARIATIONS

>>> Pizza toppings:

Try experimenting with different toppings, including:

Tomato sauce, sliced cooked chestnuts, crumbled blue cheese, chunks of cooked herb and pork sausage and sage.

Slices of Tallegio cheese, thin slices of cooked potato, prosciutto and rosemary (omit the tomato sauce).

Tomato sauce, prawns/shrimp, courgette/zucchini, basil, mozzarella, chilli oil and topped with rocket/arugula after cooking.

Tomato sauce, chorizo, black olives, jalapeños and ricotta.

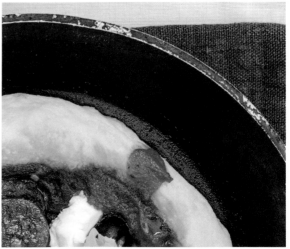

SAUCES

A sauce can make or break a meal. For me, the perfect sauce helps to unify and lift a plate of food that may be dry or dull without, rather than overshadow and swamp a good dish. I hope you'll agree that this collection of sauces all fit into the first camp, plus they are all versatile.

The Tomato Basil Sauce is an obvious choice with pasta or on top of a pizza, but it also makes a good base for hearty soups and stews. Try adding capers, spices or make it more substantial with the addition of red or green lentils and/or vegetables. Likewise, the vibrant Spanish red pepper Romesco Sauce can double up as a dip, while the Lemon Aioli can be flavoured with fresh herbs such as dill, basil or chives, or enlivened with chilli sauce or sriracha instead of lemon.

Gravy is a must-have recipe in most cooks' repertoires and this creamy version is no exception. For a more robust onion gravy, omit the cream and use red wine instead, adding 1 teaspoon yeast extract or nutritional yeast flakes.

››› Tomato basil sauce

Heat 2 tbsp olive oil and 2 finely chopped large garlic cloves in a saucepan over a low heat and cook gently for 1 minute. Add 2 x 400g/14oz cans chopped tomatoes, 1 tbsp tomato purée/paste and 1 tsp sugar. Stir well until combined, then add 1 large bunch of basil (leaves and stalks). Bring to a gentle boil, then turn the heat down to low and simmer for 15–20 minutes, part-covered, until reduced and thickened. Remove the basil and season with salt and pepper to taste.

››› Lemon aioli

To make this garlicky mayonnaise-type sauce, grind 1 small garlic clove with ½ tsp sea salt to a paste in a pestle and mortar. In a large bowl, whisk together 1 large egg yolk with 1 tsp Dijon mustard or English mustard powder until smooth and creamy. Gradually whisk in 150ml/5fl oz/scant ⅔ cup light olive oil until you achieve a mayonnaise consistency. Stir in the juice of ½ lemon and taste, adding more salt if needed. For an extra lemony aioli, stir in 2 tsp finely grated lemon zest.

»»» Romesco sauce

This roasted red pepper sauce can be served as a dip or on creamy polenta, with pasta or as a base of a bean stew. Preheat the oven to 180°C/350°F/Gas 4. Put 30g/1oz/scant ¼ cup each of blanched almonds and hazelnuts in a large roasting pan and toast for 12–15 minutes, turning once, then leave to cool. Turn the oven up to 220°C/425°F/Gas 7. Brush 1 large pepper with olive oil, put it in the roasting pan and roast for 20 minutes, then add 1 onion, cut into wedges, and 2 tomatoes, both tossed in olive oil, into the oven and roast for 20 minutes.

Ten minutes before the vegetables are ready, brush 1 slice of country-style bread with oil and bake in the oven until crisp. Put the roasted pepper in a bowl, cover with cling film/plastic wrap and leave for 5 minutes before peeling and removing the seeds.

Grind the toasted nuts in a mini food processor or using a pestle and mortar until a coarse crumb-like texture. Roughly chop the toasted bread and add to the food processor with the roasted pepper, tomatoes, onion, 2 tbsp extra virgin olive oil and 2 tsp white wine vinegar. Add 1 crushed garlic clove and 2 tbsp water and process to a slightly chunky sauce-like consistency. Season with salt and 1 tsp dried chilli/hot pepper flakes. Stir in extra water to make a looser sauce, if desired.

»»» Creamy onion gravy

This is delicious with nut roasts, pies and roasted winter root vegetables. To make the gravy, melt 2 tbsp butter in a saucepan over a medium-low heat. Add 1 large finely chopped onion and cook for 10 minutes, part-covered, until softened. Add 2 tbsp plain/all purpose flour and stir the paste constantly for 2 minutes to cook out the flour. Add 150ml/5fl oz/scant ⅔ cup dry white wine and cook for 5 minutes, stirring, until reduced and there is no aroma of alcohol. Gradually stir in 500ml/17fl oz/generous 2 cups vegetable stock and simmer for 10–15 minutes, or until reduced and thickened. Using a stick/immersion blender, blend the gravy until smooth, then stir in 2 tbsp double/heavy cream. Season and reheat just before serving.

Hand-raised mushroom pie

SERVES ⟫⟫ **6–8**

Preparation time ⟩ 40 minutes

Cooking time ⟩ 1 hour

25g/1oz/1 cup dried porcini
    mushrooms

40g/1½oz/2½ tbsp butter

2 leeks, finely chopped

4 garlic cloves, finely chopped

2 tbsp thyme leaves or 1 tbsp dried

1 tbsp chopped rosemary

500g/1lb 2oz forestière or chestnut/
    cremini mushrooms, finely chopped

2 carrots, finely grated

2 tbsp light soy sauce

200g/7oz/1⅓ cups day-old fresh
    breadcrumbs

2 tbsp crème fraîche

sea salt and freshly ground black
    pepper

⟫⟫ Hot-water crust pastry

50g/1¾oz/3½ tbsp butter, cut into
    pieces, plus extra for greasing

550g/1lb 4oz/scant 4¼ cups plain/
    all-purpose flour, plus extra
    for dusting

1 tsp salt

125g/4½oz vegetable fat, cut into
    small pieces

1 egg, lightly beaten, to glaze

This impressive pie has a hot-water crust pastry case – so it looks similar to the classic English pork pie – and is filled with a combination of mushrooms, herbs and vegetables, with or without the addition of the ham hock option on the next page. Don't be put off by the pastry – it is surprisingly straightforward to make as long as you work with it when it's slightly warm and malleable. The beauty of this substantial pie is that it is equally good served warm for a Sunday lunch or celebratory meal with all the trimmings as it is cold for a picnic or as part of a buffet lunch.

⟫⟫ To make the pie filling, put the dried porcini in a bowl and cover with just-boiled water. Leave for 20 minutes to soften, then drain well (reserving the soaking liquid for another recipe). Squeeze out any excess water and roughly chop the porcini.

⟫⟫ Heat the butter in a large sauté pan over a medium-low heat and fry the leeks for 3 minutes until softened. Increase the heat to medium, add the porcini, garlic, thyme, rosemary, mushrooms, carrots and soy sauce and cook for another 5–7 minutes, stirring regularly, until the vegetables are tender and there is no trace of liquid. Stir in the breadcrumbs followed by the crème fraîche, then season generously with salt and pepper. Transfer the mixture to a bowl to cool.

⟫⟫ Meanwhile, make the pastry. Preheat the oven to 200°C/400°F/Gas 6 and lightly grease a 20cm/8in deep springform cake pan. Put the flour and salt in a large mixing bowl and make a well in the middle. Heat the butter and vegetable fat with 200ml/7fl oz/scant 1 cup water in a saucepan, stirring until it comes to the boil. Pour the mixture into the flour and mix with a wooden spoon and then your fingers until it comes together into a ball of dough. Tip the dough onto a lightly floured work surface.

⟫⟫ Working quickly, cut off one-third of the pastry, cover and set aside. Roll out the remaining pastry and use to line the prepared pan, pressing it into the base and up the sides. Spoon the mushroom mixture into the pan. Roll out the remaining pastry to make a lid. Dampen the edge of the pastry case, put the lid on top and trim any excess. Press the edges together to seal and crimp neatly.

⟫⟫ Brush the top of the pie with the egg and make a couple of steam holes in the middle. Cut leaves from the pastry trimmings to decorate the top of the pie and brush with a little more egg. Bake for 50 minutes, or until the pastry is crisp and golden, placing foil over the top of the pie if it browns too quickly. Leave to stand on a wire rack for 10 minutes before removing from the pan. Serve warm or cold, cut into wedges.

PART-TIME VARIATION

››› Ham hock and mushroom pie

Prepare a half quantity of the mushroom mixture following the instructions on the previous page, then leave to cool. Meanwhile, put **400g/14oz thinly sliced or shredded, cooked ham hock**, **3 tbsp crème fraîche**, **1 heaped tsp English mustard**, **¼ tsp freshly grated nutmeg** and **4 tbsp chopped flat-leaf parsley leaves** in a large mixing bowl and season with salt and pepper. Mix together until combined.

To assemble the pie, follow the instructions for making the pastry as described previously and use to line the pan as instructed. Spoon the ham mixture into the pastry case in an even layer. Top with the mushroom mixture and spread it out evenly over the ham. To finish making the pie, top with the pastry lid and bake as described before.

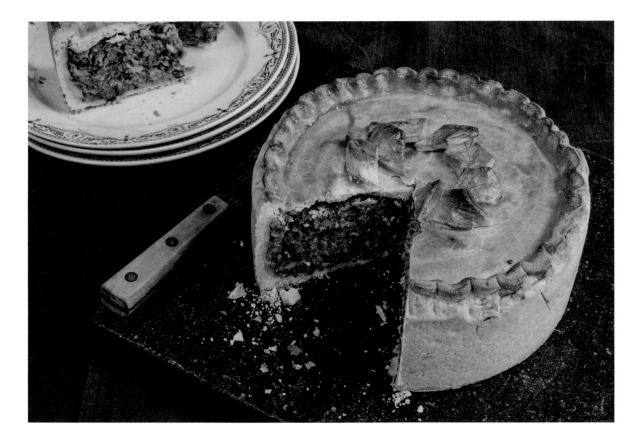

Pumpkin <u>AND</u> cashew wellington <u>WITH</u> parsnip crisps

SERVES ⟩⟩⟩ **4–6**

Preparation time ⟩ 25 minutes
Cooking time ⟩ 65 minutes

850g/1lb 14oz pumpkin or butternut
   squash, skin removed, deseeded
   and cut into bite-size chunks
2 tbsp olive oil
1 red chilli, deseeded and finely
   chopped (optional)
175g/6oz/scant 1½ cups cashew nuts
1 large onion, chopped
3 garlic cloves, chopped
5 tbsp chopped sage leaves
3 tbsp chopped rosemary
55g/2oz/scant 1 cup day-old fresh
   breadcrumbs
200g/7oz/1½ cups cooked, peeled
   chestnuts, finely chopped
2 eggs, lightly beaten
1 tbsp yeast extract
flour, for dusting
400g/14oz puff pastry
sea salt and freshly ground black
   pepper
1 recipe quantity Creamy Onion Gravy,
   to serve (see page 201), (optional)

⟩⟩⟩ Parsnip crisps

1 parsnip, cut into ribbons using
   a vegetable peeler
1 tbsp olive oil

Perfect as an alternative Sunday roast or a Christmas meal centrepiece, this pie has a layer of orange-fleshed pumpkin running down the middle, which is sandwiched between a toasted cashew and sage stuffing. The whole thing is then wrapped in puff pastry and baked until flaky and golden. If you want to make the sausage and herb wellington variation on the next page to serve at the same time, you could make smaller parcels containing both filling options. Either way, serve with roast potatoes and all your favourite accompaniments.

⟩⟩⟩ Preheat the oven to 200°C/400°F/Gas 6. Toss the pumpkin in half the olive oil, then spread out in a large roasting pan and season with salt and pepper. Roast for 25 minutes until tender but not coloured. Transfer to a bowl and mash with the back of a fork to a chunky purée. Stir in the chilli, if using, then leave to cool.

⟩⟩⟩ Meanwhile, put the cashews in a separate roasting pan and toast in the bottom of the oven for 8 minutes, or until starting to colour.

⟩⟩⟩ While the pumpkin and cashews are cooking, heat the remaining oil in a large frying pan over a medium heat. Add the onion and cook for 7 minutes until softened, stirring often. Add the garlic and cook for another minute. ⟩

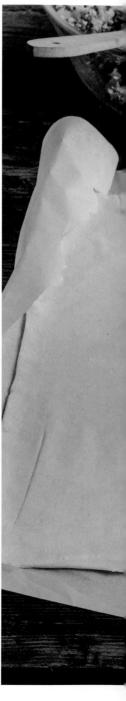

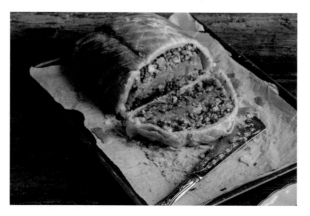

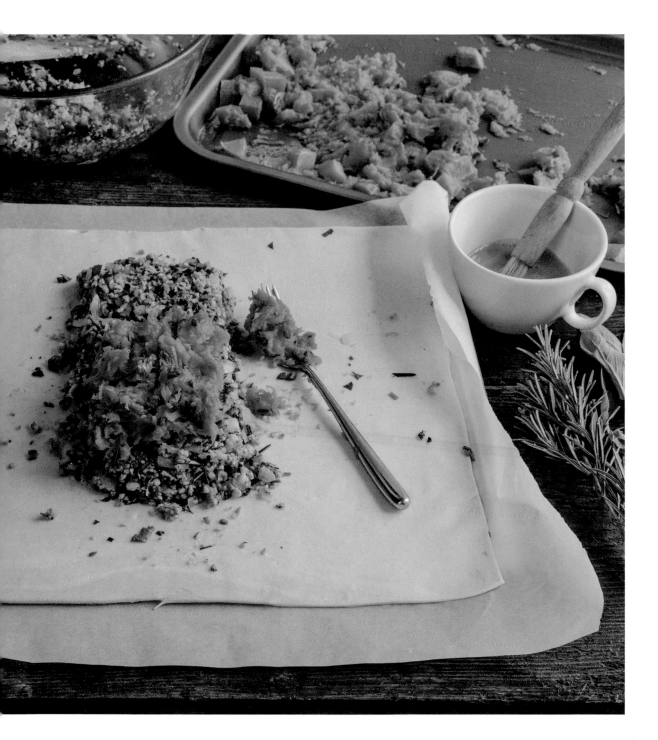

⟩⟩⟩ Transfer the onion mixture to a bowl and stir in the herbs, breadcrumbs, chestnuts, one of the beaten eggs and the yeast extract. Finely chop the cashews, then add to the bowl and stir well until combined. Season generously with pepper.

⟩⟩⟩ Lightly dust a work surface with flour and roll out the pastry on a piece of baking paper to a 34 × 30cm/13½ × 12in rectangle. Spoon half of the cashew mixture down the middle of the shortest length of the pastry, in a strip about 12cm/4½in wide, leaving a gap either side and at each end of the pastry. Spoon the pumpkin mixture on top in an even layer, then follow with the remaining cashew mixture. Brush the edges of the pastry with a little of the remaining egg and fold them over the filling to meet in the middle. Trim any excess pastry and press the edges together to seal. Make diagonal slashes in the top of the pastry and fold in the ends to seal in the filling.

⟩⟩⟩ Carefully, lift the wellington using the paper to a non-stick roasting pan, and brush the top with the remaining beaten egg. Cut down any excess baking paper and bake for 35–40 minutes until the pastry is golden.

⟩⟩⟩ Meanwhile, make the parsnip crisps. Toss the parsnips in the oil, season with salt and pepper, then put in a roasting pan. Roast at the same time as the wellington for 15–20 minutes until crisp and light golden. Serve the wellington cut into thick slices, topped with the parsnip crisps and with the Creamy Onion Gravy by the side, if you like.

PART-TIME VARIATION
⟩⟩⟩ Sausage and herb wellington

Prepare the wellington as described on page 204, replacing the cashews with 300g/10½oz good-quality herb and pork sausagemeat. Stir the sausagemeat into the onion and herb mixture with 25g/1oz/⅓ cup day-old fresh breadcrumbs, 150g/5½oz/1¼ cups finely chopped cooked chestnuts and 1 tbsp yeast extract (omitting the egg). Assemble the wellington as described, placing a layer of the pumpkin purée between the sausagemeat stuffing, then bake for 40–45 minutes. Serve with the parsnip crisps, as described above.

Moroccan-style marrow
WITH baba ganoush

If stuffed marrow sounds a bit 'old-school' vegetarian, ditch any pre-conceived ideas as this lifts the humble vegetable to new heights. For starters, the marrow is roasted separately from its filling until it starts to caramelize. This also means that there is little risk of the bulgur wheat, date and pistachio stuffing drying out. Secondly, it comes with a marrow baba ganoush made from the scooped out flesh, so nothing goes to waste.

⟫⟫⟫ Preheat the oven to 200°C/400°F/Gas 6. Scoop out and discard the seeds of the marrow using a teaspoon, then brush the flesh all over with 1 tablespoon of the olive oil. Place the marrow in a roasting pan, cut-side up, and roast for 30 minutes, turning once, until tender and the flesh starts to turn golden.

⟫⟫⟫ At the same time, put the pistachios in a roasting pan and roast in the bottom of the oven for 8 minutes, or until starting to colour. Leave the nuts to cool, then chop roughly.

⟫⟫⟫ Meanwhile, put the bulgur in a pan and pour enough water over to cover by 2cm/¾in. Stir in the turmeric and bring to the boil, then turn the heat down to low and simmer for 15 minutes, covered, until very tender. Drain the bulgur and transfer to a bowl.

⟫⟫⟫ While the marrow and bulgur are cooking, heat the remaining oil in a large frying pan over a medium heat. Add the onion and cook for 7 minutes until softened, then add the garlic, dates, preserved lemon, cardamom, ginger and chilli/hot pepper flakes and cook for 2 minutes, or until the dates start to soften. Stir the onion mixture into the bulgur with the herbs and season with salt and pepper.

⟫⟫⟫ When the marrow is ready, make the baba ganoush. Scoop out most of the marrow flesh leaving a 1cm/½in shell. Transfer the flesh to a beaker with the garlic, yogurt, tahini and lemon juice and blend with a stick/immersion blender to a smooth purée. Season to taste and leave to one side.

⟫⟫⟫ Pile the bulgur mixture into the marrow shell, scatter the pistachios over the top and serve with the baba ganoush.

SERVES ⟫⟫⟫ **4**

Preparation time ⟩ 20 minutes
Cooking time ⟩ 30 minutes

1 marrow, about 28cm/11¼in in length, halved lengthways
3 tbsp extra virgin olive oil, plus extra for drizzling
55g/2oz/heaped ⅓ cup pistachio nuts
100g/3½oz/heaped ½ cup bulgur wheat
1 tsp turmeric
1 large onion, finely chopped
2 large garlic cloves, finely chopped
55g/2oz/scant ½ cup pitted dried dates, chopped
1 tbsp finely chopped Cheat's Preserved Lemons (see page 165), or shop-bought
seeds from 2 cardamom pods, ground
1 tsp ground ginger
½ tsp dried chilli/hot pepper flakes
2 large handfuls of chopped coriander/ cilantro leaves
1 large handful of chopped mint leaves
sea salt and freshly ground black pepper

⟫⟫⟫ Baba ganoush
1 garlic clove, halved
4 tbsp plain yogurt
1 tbsp tahini
2 tbsp lemon juice

Butternut squash-stuffed pasta shells WITH Tallegio cheese

SERVES ⟩⟩⟩ 4

Preparation time ⟩ 20 minutes
Cooking time ⟩ 45 minutes

1 small butternut squash, peeled,
    deseeded and cubed (about
    500g/1lb 2oz net weight)
400g/14oz large dried pasta shells
2 tbsp olive oil
40g/1½oz/2½ tbsp butter
40g/1½oz/⅓ cup plain/
    all-purpose flour
800ml/28fl oz/3½ cups warm milk
300g/10½oz Tallegio cheese, rind
    discarded, cut into pieces
3 garlic cloves, finely chopped
2 tbsp finely chopped rosemary
40g/1½oz/⅔ cup finely grated
    Parmesan cheese
3 tbsp toasted chopped walnuts
    (see method on page 22)

The beauty of this rich, satisfying dish is that it can be prepared in advance and then assembled and cooked in 30 minutes, making it an ideal meal for an informal gathering. The same goes for the Chicken, Leek and Sage variation on the next page. Look for large pasta shells, which are perfect for stuffing and look attractive, too.

⟩⟩⟩ Steam or boil the squash for 10–15 minutes until tender. Meanwhile, cook the pasta in plenty of boiling salted water for 10 minutes until just al dente, but not quite cooked. Drain, return the pasta to the pan and toss in half the oil to prevent the shells sticking together.

⟩⟩⟩ Preheat the oven to 200°C/400°F/Gas 6. While the pasta and squash are cooking, melt the butter in a medium-size pan over a medium-low heat, add the flour and cook the paste for 2 minutes, stirring. Gradually add the milk, whisking continuously, until thickened to a white sauce consistency, about 5 minutes. Stir in the Tallegio until melted, then season with salt and pepper. Leave to one side.

⟩⟩⟩ Heat the remaining oil in a frying pan over a medium-low heat and fry the garlic and rosemary for 1 minute until softened. Stir in the cooked squash, season with salt and pepper, then remove from the heat. Add 2 tablespoons hot water to the pan and roughly mash the squash to a coarse purée.

⟩⟩⟩ Spoon a little of the Tallegio sauce into the bottom of a large ovenproof dish. Arrange the pasta shells in the dish and fill each one with the squash purée. Pour the remaining Tallegio sauce over the shells to cover and sprinkle with some of the Parmesan. Cover with foil and bake for 30 minutes, or until the pasta is tender. Serve sprinkled with the remaining Parmesan and toasted walnuts.

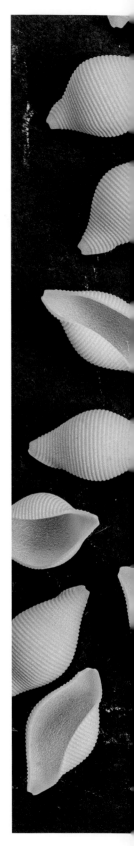

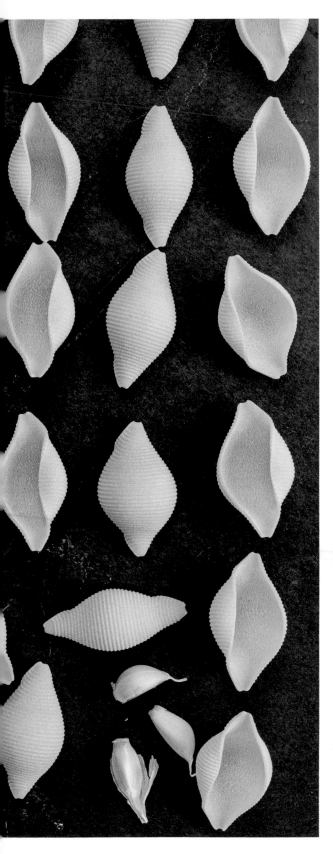

PART-TIME VARIATION
»»» Chicken, leek and sage stuffed pasta

As an alternative to the squash, heat 1 tbsp olive oil in a frying pan and fry **500g/1lb 2oz skinless, boneless chicken breasts**, cut into pieces, for 5 minutes until browned all over. Remove the chicken from the pan with a slotted spoon and finely chop. Add **1 finely chopped leek** and **2 tbsp chopped sage** to the pan, adding a little extra oil, if needed. Cook the leek for 5 minutes until softened, then return the chicken to the pan, remove from the heat and stir until combined.

Fill the part-cooked pasta shells with the chicken mixture, cover with the Tallegio sauce and bake as described on the previous page.

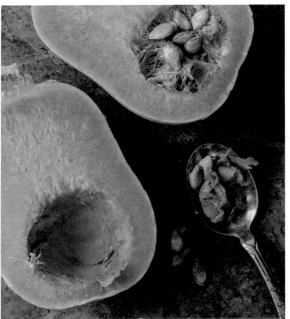

Halloumi WITH aubergine caviar AND lentils

SERVES ››› 4

Preparation time › 20 minutes
Cooking time › 55 minutes

finely grated zest and juice of 2 limes

3 tbsp extra virgin olive oil, plus extra
    for brushing and drizzling

400g/14oz halloumi cheese, rinsed and
    patted dry, cut into 12 x 1cm/½in
    thick slices

2 aubergines/eggplants

3 large garlic cloves, finely chopped

300g/10½oz/heaped 1½ cups
    Puy lentils

2 tsp vegetable bouillon powder

2 handfuls of roughly chopped
    coriander/cilantro leaves

2 tbsp light tahini

1 long red chilli, deseeded and
    thinly sliced

sea salt and freshly ground black
    pepper

For convenience, both the aubergine/eggplant caviar and the coriander/cilantro-infused lentils can be made in advance and are equally good served at room temperature as they are warm. Not so the halloumi, which is best cooked just before serving as it is prone to turn rubbery when cold. If you have any leftover aubergine/eggplant caviar, try serving it as a dip with warm pitta or flatbread.

››› Preheat the oven to 220°C/425°F/Gas 7. While the oven is heating, mix together the lime juice and zest with 1 tablespoon of the olive oil in a shallow dish. Add the halloumi, spoon the lime marinade over and leave to one side.

››› Put the aubergines/eggplants in a roasting pan, prick all over with a skewer, brush with oil and roast for 45 minutes, or until very tender.

››› While the aubergines/eggplants are roasting, heat the remaining oil in a saucepan over a medium-low heat. Add 2 of the garlic cloves and sauté for 1 minute until softened but not coloured. Add the lentils and cover with 750ml/26fl oz/generous 3¼ cups water. Bring to the boil, then turn the heat down and simmer for 20 minutes, part-covered. Stir in the bouillon powder, then simmer for a further 10 minutes until the lentils are tender. Remove from the heat, stir in the coriander/cilantro, season, cover with a lid and leave to one side.

››› To finish the aubergine/eggplant caviar, cut in half lengthways and scoop out the flesh into a blender, discarding any overly seedy bits. Add the tahini, half the lime juice marinade from the halloumi and the remaining garlic and blend until smooth and creamy. (For a coarser purée, mash with a potato masher or the back of a fork.) Season with salt and pepper to taste, adding more of the lime juice marinade if needed.

››› To prepare the halloumi, heat a griddle/grill pan over a high heat then brush with oil. Remove the halloumi from any remaining marinade and griddle/grill in two batches for 3–4 minutes, turning once, until slightly blackened in places.

››› To serve, spoon the lentils into large, shallow serving bowls, top with a good spoonful of the aubergine/eggplant caviar and then the halloumi, drizzle a little extra oil over and scatter with the chilli.

Aubergine AND olive stifado WITH baked feta

Here are a meat-free and a classic lamb version of the Greek stew, stifado. Either makes a nourishing, comforting meal, perfect for sharing with family and friends. They can happily be made in advance and then reheated when needed, which seems to heighten the flavour of the stew, with its warming hint of cinnamon and cloves.

>>> Cook the potatoes in plenty of boiling, salted water for 10 minutes, or until almost cooked, then drain and leave to one side. Meanwhile, heat the oil in a large casserole over a medium-low heat. Add the shallots and cook for 5 minutes, covered and stirring occasionally, until tender. Add the aubergine/eggplant and cook for another 8 minutes, stirring occasionally, until tender. Stir in the garlic and spices, then pour in the wine and let it bubble away for about 5 minutes until reduced and there is no aroma of alcohol.

>>> Add the vinegar, passata/sieved tomatoes, tomato purée/paste, oregano, olives, beans, cooked potatoes and 150ml/5fl oz/scant ⅔ cup water. Bring to the boil, then turn the heat down and simmer for 20 minutes, part-covered, or until the sauce has reduced and thickened. Add more water if the sauce is too dry or remove the lid if it needs to reduce more. Season with salt and pepper to taste.

>>> While the stifado is cooking, preheat the oven to 180°C/350°F/Gas 4. Place the feta in the middle of a piece of foil. Sprinkle with oregano and drizzle a little oil over the top. Gather the edges of the foil together to make a parcel and place in a baking pan. Bake for 12–15 minutes until softened. Serve the stifado topped with the feta, extra oregano and a drizzle of olive oil. Serve with orzo or crusty bread.

PART-TIME VARIATION
>>> Lamb and butter bean stifado

Heat 1 tbsp olive oil in a large casserole over a medium heat and cook 1 large sliced onion for 8 minutes, covered, until softened. Remove from the casserole with a slotted spoon and brown 750g/1lb 10oz cubed shoulder of lamb in two batches for 5 minutes. Preheat the oven to 170°C/325°F/Gas 3.

Return the onions and lamb to the casserole with 3 sliced garlic cloves, 1 small cinnamon stick, 7 cloves and 1 tbsp oregano leaves. Stir well and add 175ml/6fl oz/scant ¾ cup red wine, 2 tbsp red wine vinegar, 500g/1lb 2oz carton passata and 2 tbsp tomato purée/paste. Add 150ml/5fl oz/scant ⅔ cup water and 400g/14oz can butter beans. Bring to the boil, cover, and put in the oven for 1½ hours or until the lamb is tender. Serve with orzo or crusty bread.

SERVES >>> **4**

Preparation time ⟩ 15 minutes
Cooking time ⟩ 40 minutes

300g/10½oz new potatoes, scrubbed and quartered
3 tbsp extra virgin olive oil, plus extra for drizzling
350g/12oz shallots or baby onions, halved if large
1 large aubergine/eggplant, cubed
3 garlic cloves, finely chopped
1 small cinnamon stick
7 cloves
175ml/6fl oz/scant ¾ cup red wine
2 tbsp red wine vinegar
500ml/17fl oz/2 cups passata/sieved tomatoes
2 tbsp tomato purée/paste
1 heaped tbsp oregano leaves, plus extra sprigs, for sprinkling and serving
85g/3oz/scant 1 cup pitted black olives
400g/14oz can butter beans, drained and rinsed
sea salt and freshly ground black pepper
orzo pasta or crusty bread, to serve

>>> Baked feta
300g/10½oz block of sheep's feta cheese
1 tsp oregano leaves

Fresh summer lasagne
<u>WITH</u> herb oil

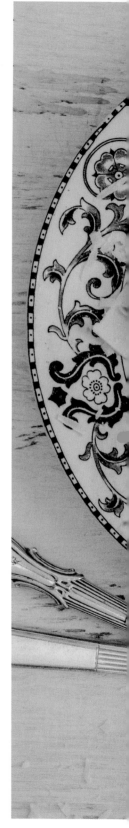

SERVES ⟩⟩⟩ 4

Preparation time ⟩ 30 minutes
Cooking time ⟩ 30 minutes

4 courgettes/zucchini, halved crossways
    and each half cut lengthways into
    ribbons using a vegetable peeler
12 baby spring onions/scallions,
    trimmed
2 tbsp olive oil
250g/9oz/2 cups shelled broad/fava
    beans
200g/7oz runner beans, thinly sliced
    diagonally
200g/7oz baby spinach leaves
2 garlic cloves, finely chopped
finely grated zest and juice of 1 lemon
6 tbsp double/heavy cream
8 fresh lasagne sheets
80g/2¾oz hard sheep's cheese or
    Parmesan cheese, pared into
    shavings
1 handful of pumpkin seeds, toasted
    (see method on page 71)

⟩⟩⟩ Herb oil

6 tbsp extra virgin olive oil
1 small garlic clove, halved
1 large handful of basil leaves
3 tbsp lemon thyme leaves
2 tbsp snipped chives, plus extra whole
    chives, to serve
a squeeze of lemon juice
sea salt and freshly ground black
    pepper

This is lasagne, but not as you know it as it really couldn't be more different to the classic version. The 'open' lasagne makes the most of wonderful seasonal vegetables and is a great summery meal when you don't want anything too heavy. The herb oil uses a combination of basil, chives and lemon thyme, but do try any fresh herbs that you have to hand – parsley, oregano and basil are good, too.

⟩⟩⟩ To make the herb oil, put all the ingredients in a blender and blend to a slightly coarse purée. Season with salt and pepper to taste, then leave to one side.

⟩⟩⟩ Put the courgettes/zucchini and spring onions/scallions in a large bowl, pour half of the olive oil over, season and toss with your hands until the vegetables are coated in the oil. Heat a large griddle/grill pan over a high heat and griddle/grill the courgettes/zucchini in batches for 8 minutes, turning once. Keep the cooked courgettes/zucchini warm in a low oven. Next, griddle the spring onions/scallions in two batches for 3 minutes, turning once. Keep all the cooked vegetables warm in the oven.

⟩⟩⟩ While the vegetables are griddling, steam the broad/fava beans and runner beans for 3–4 minutes until tender. Refresh under cold running water, then pop the broad beans out of their grey shells to reveal the bright green beans inside. Leave to one side.

⟩⟩⟩ Heat the remaining olive oil in a large sauté pan over a medium heat. Add the spinach and cook for 3 minutes, turning it with tongs, until almost wilted. Add the garlic and cook for one more minute. Next, add the lemon zest and juice and the cooked beans and turn until combined. Turn the heat down to low, pour in the cream, season and heat briefly until warmed through.

⟩⟩⟩ Meanwhile, cook the lasagne sheets in plenty of boiling salted water, following the instructions on the pack, until al dente. Drain and put a sheet of lasagne on each serving plate. Divide the spinach mixture between the plates.

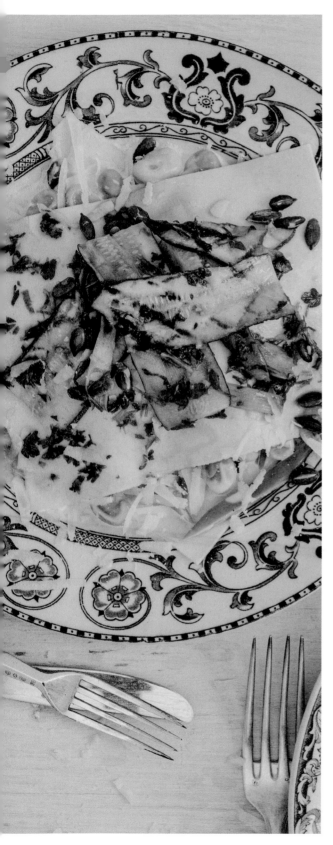

Top with half the cheese and another layer of lasagne. Next, arrange the griddled courgettes/zucchini and spring onions/scallions on top of the second sheet of lasagne. Drizzle over the herb oil and finally scatter the pumpkin seeds, whole chives and the remaining cheese on top.

PART-TIME VARIATION
⟩⟩⟩ Seafood lasagne with herb oil

First make the herb oil as described on the previous page, replacing the thyme with **3 tbsp oregano leaves.**

Replace the courgettes/zucchini with **400g/14oz raw, peeled large prawns/jumbo shrimp.** Start by griddling/grilling the spring onions/scallions and cooking the beans as described on the previous page.

Cook the spinach, as described before, for 2 minutes then add the prawns/shrimp with the garlic and cook for another minute before adding the lemon zest and juice and cooked beans. Pour in the cream and heat through. Cook the lasagne and serve as described above, omitting the pumpkin seeds.

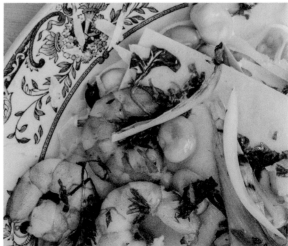

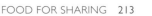

Wild garlic AND asparagus filo tart

SERVES ⟫⟫ **4–6**

Preparation time ⟫ 25 minutes
Cooking time ⟫ 40 minutes

3 tbsp olive oil
5 shallots or 1 large onion (about
    200g/7oz total weight), finely
    chopped
250g/9oz bunch asparagus, trimmed
1 large garlic clove, finely chopped
6 sheets of filo/phyllo pastry
150ml/5fl oz/scant ⅔ cup double/
    heavy cream
2 large eggs, beaten
55g/2oz/¾ cup finely grated Parmesan
    cheese
2 large handfuls of finely chopped wild
    garlic or chives (flowers reserved,
    if any)
1 tbsp chopped oregano or marjoram
    leaves
sea salt and freshly ground black
    pepper
1 recipe quantity Lemon Aioli,
    to serve (see page 200)

The season for wild garlic coincides perfectly with that of asparagus, so it seems only natural to partner the two in this springtime tart. For other times of the year, you could try chopped chives, spring onions/ scallions or steamed leeks instead of the wild garlic, while long-stem broccoli or spinach would work well in place of the asparagus, too. The springform cake pan is a must as it makes the tart so much easier to serve, especially when using fragile filo/phyllo pastry.

⟫⟫ Heat 1 tablespoon of the olive oil in a large frying pan over a medium heat. Add the shallots and fry for 5 minutes, stirring occasionally, until softened.

⟫⟫ While the shallots are cooking, cut the tip off each asparagus stem, about 2.5cm/1in from the top. Peel the stems and finely slice into rounds. Add the asparagus tips and stems to the pan with the shallots and garlic and cook for 2–3 minutes until the asparagus is almost tender, then leave to cool.

⟫⟫ Preheat the oven to 200°C/400°F/Gas 6. Lightly grease a 23cm/9in springform cake pan with a little of the remaining oil. Place a sheet of filo/phyllo in the pan, gently pressing it into the base and up the side, leaving any surplus pastry to overhang the top. Brush the pastry with a little of the oil and top with a second sheet of pastry, then continue until you have six layers of filo/phyllo.

⟫⟫ Whisk together the cream and eggs, season with salt and pepper and stir in the Parmesan cheese, wild garlic and asparagus mixture. Pour the mixture into the pastry case and sprinkle with the oregano. Fold the overhanging pastry back over the filling, scrunching it as you go to give a 2.5cm/1in wide edge to the top of the tart. Brush the pastry with a little oil and bake for 25–30 minutes until the pastry is golden and the filling is set.

⟫⟫ Leave to rest for 5 minutes, then carefully remove the tart from the pan – leave it on the base, if that's easier. Serve warm with the lemon aioli on the side.

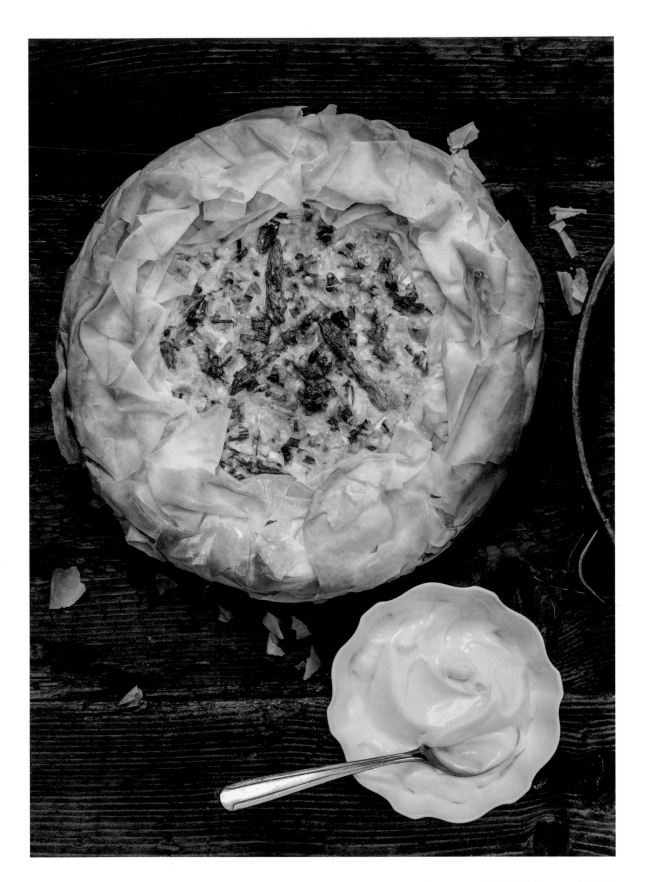

Planning ahead

The menu plans on the following pages give you plenty of ideas of how to combine the recipes found in this book. The plans have been created to suit various eating occasions, whether you're looking for a week's worth of healthy vegetarian meals, a special meal for friends and family that can be made in advance, or suggestions for a part-time vegetarian week's worth of meal ideas that includes meat and fish in small amounts, but is predominantly veggie.

I always find it easier at the start of the week to mentally plan what we'll be eating as a family throughout the week to come, so there's a balance and variety of ingredients and plenty of variation in terms of taste, texture and colour. So if pasta is on the menu for dinner one evening, then it will be rice, potatoes, pulses or other grains on subsequent nights. Similarly, the source of protein varies – whether it be tofu, eggs, cheese or lentils – along with the origin of the dish, so that means we may eat something that is inspired by Indian, Thai or Chinese cuisines one evening and Italian, English or French the next.

Now, I'm not saying that we all have to eat in this way, but the crux of these menus is to make planning ahead that much easier, so when time is tight they help you mix-and-match the recipes in the book. They're not meant to be prescriptive, merely suggestive, so feel free to swap any recipe ideas that don't fit in with personal or family likes or dislikes. After all, cooking (and, of course, eating) is all about enjoyment and nourishing ourselves, rather than punishment and going without.

As mentioned earlier in the book, many of the vegetarian recipes have what is called a 'Part-time Variation'. These sub-recipes are meat-, poultry- or seafood-based, so in keeping with the title of the book, there are also menus for those who want ideas of how to easily adapt a vegetarian meal into one that will appeal to meat and fish eaters as well. These menus would be perfect for when you have a range of eating preferences at one mealtime, which can be a bit of a headache but at least you come well prepared.

FAMILY VEGETARIAN WEEK

MONDAY
- **Breakfast**: Toast with Almond and Cashew Butter (see page 41)
- **Lunch**: Halloumi Hash (see page 50)
- **Dinner**: Quinoa and Borlotti Burgers (see page 130)

TUESDAY
- **Breakfast**: Quinoa Granola (see page 20)
- **Lunch**: Mung Bean Humous with Sesame Pitta Crisps (see page 71)
- **Dinner**: Tomato, Olive and Mozzarella Rice (see page 124)

WEDNESDAY
- **Breakfast**: Nut Butter and Cinnamon Smoothie (see page 18)
- **Lunch**: Smoked Paprika, Tomato and Herb Scramble (see page 47)
- **Dinner**: Orecchiette with Pea and Mint Pesto (see page 132)

THURSDAY
- **Breakfast**: Orange Bircher Muesli (see page 19)
- **Lunch**: Courgette, Mint and Feta Fritters (see page 70)
- **Dinner**: Kosheri (see page 52)

FRIDAY
- **Breakfast**: Porridge with Apricot and Vanilla Spread (see page 40)
- **Lunch**: Char Sui Tofu Cups (see page 80)
- **Dinner**: Okonomiyaki (see page 114)

SATURDAY
- **Breakfast**: Coconut and Cardamom Pancakes with Mango (see page 32)
- **Lunch**: Sushi Cones with Pickled Ginger (see page 186)
- **Dinner**: Slow-rise Pan Pizzas (see page 198)

SUNDAY
- **Brunch**: Nut Butter and Cinnamon Smoothie (see page 18) and Breakfast Tortillas (see page 46)
- **Dinner**: Pumpkin and Cashew Wellington with Parsnip Crisps (see page 204)

PART-TIME VEGETARIAN WEEK

MONDAY
- **Breakfast**: Orange Bircher Muesli (see page 19)
- **Lunch**: Saag Aloo Wraps (see page 86)
- **Dinner**: Mexican Eggs with Corn Chips (see page 87)

TUESDAY
- **Breakfast**: Quinoa Granola (see page 20)
- **Lunch**: Caper, Crumb and Lemon Linguine (see page 133)
- **Dinner**: Lamb with White Bean Mash (see page 105)

WEDNESDAY
- **Breakfast**: Nut Butter and Cinnamon Smoothie (see page 18)
- **Lunch**: Chicken Panzanella (see page 65)
- **Dinner**: Aubergine and Olive Stifado with Baked Feta (see page 211)

THURSDAY
- **Breakfast**: Ham and Mozzarella Toasts (see page 36)
- **Lunch**: Smoked Paprika, Tomato and Herb Scramble (see page 47)
- **Dinner**: Roasted Vegetables with Skorthalia (see page 104)

FRIDAY
- **Breakfast**: Egg Pots with Asparagus Dippers (see page 44)
- **Lunch**: Sour Cherry, Red Quinoa and Spiced Almond Salad (see page 60)
- **Dinner**: Lentil and Apricot Pilaf with Spiced Cauliflower (see page 122)

SATURDAY
- **Breakfast**: Pikelets with Pear and Ginger Compôte (see page 30)
- **Lunch**: White Bean Soup with Cumin Carrot Mash (see page 96)
- **Dinner**: Chorizo and Prawn/Shrimp Tomato Rice (see page 124)

SUNDAY
- **Brunch**: Quinoa Granola (see page 20); Seed and Spice Soda Bread with Smoked Mackerel Pâté (see page 23)
- **Dinner**: Mushroom and Brie Pancakes with Cider Sauce (see page 168)

7-DAY HEALTHY WEEK

MONDAY
- **Breakfast**: Orange Bircher Muesli (see page 19)
- **Lunch**: Avocado Gazpacho (see page 56), or Udon Noodle Broth (see page 59)
- **Dinner**: Chickpea Dahl with Spinach Tarka (see page 121)

TUESDAY
- **Breakfast**: Savoury Miso Porridge with Cashews (see page 22)
- **Lunch**: Mung Bean Humous with Sesame Pitta Crisps (see page 71)
- **Dinner**: Indonesian Stir-fried Rice (see page 126)

WEDNESDAY
- **Breakfast**: What's-in-the-cupboard Muesli (see page 19)
- **Lunch**: Steamed Tofu in Ginger-Soy Dressing (see page 82)
- **Dinner**: Baked Avocado with Chilli Beans (see page 120)

THURSDAY
- **Breakfast**: Nut Butter and Cinnamon Smoothie (see page 18)
- **Lunch**: Seaweed and Kamut Salad (see page 98)
- **Dinner**: Ribollita (see page 94)

FRIDAY
- **Breakfast**: What's-in-the-cupboard Muesli (see page 19)
- **Lunch**: Egg Pots with Asparagus Dippers (see page 44)
- **Dinner**: Quinoa and Borlotti Burgers (see page 130)

SATURDAY
- **Breakfast**: Quinoa Granola (see page 20)
- **Lunch**: Olive and Tomato Chickpea Pancakes (see page 34)
- **Dinner**: Aubergine Polpettine (see page 143)

SUNDAY
- **Brunch**: Nut Butter and Cinnamon Smoothie (see page 18); Home-style Baked Beans with Roasted Portabellini (see page 48)
- **Dinner**: Artichoke and Saffron Ragoût with Lemon Aioli (see page 190)

PART-TIME VEGETARIAN MEALS FOR FRIENDS

MENU 1
- Okonomiyaki (with optional Smoked Salmon variation), (see page 114)
- Asparagus and Ginger Potstickers (with optional Pork and Ginger variation), (see page 140)

MENU 2
- Roasted Pepper and Pine Nut Pissaladière (with optional Anchovy and Basil variation), (see page 151)
- Caper, Crumb and Lemon Linguine (with optional Parma Ham variation), (see page 133)

MENU 3
- Avocado Gazpacho (with optional Bresaola Crisps variation), (see page 56)
- Asparagus and Parmesan Panzanella (with optional Chicken variation), (see page 64)

MENU 4
- Salt and Szechuan Pepper Tofu (with optional Squid variation), (see page 116)
- Teriyaki Vegetables with Wakame Pickle (with optional Mackerel variation), (see page 193)

MENU 5
- Olive and Tomato Chickpea Pancakes (with optional Chicken or Prawn/Shrimp variation), (see page 34)
- Aubergine and Olive Stifado with Baked Feta (with optional Lamb and Butter Bean variation), (see page 211)

MENU 6
- Ribollita (with optional Ham Hock variation), (see page 94)
- Orecchiette with Pea and Mint Pesto (with optional Salmon variation), (see page 132)

MENUS FOR DIFFERENT OCCASIONS

ASIAN MEAL FOR SHARING
- Sushi Cones with Pickled Ginger (see page 186)
- Char Sui Tofu Cups (see page 80)
- Noodle Pot with Thai Pesto (see page 118)

SUNDAY LUNCH
- Beetroot Soup with Spiced Orange Yogurt (see page 58)
- Pumpkin and Cashew Wellington with Parsnip Crisps (see page 204)
- Pan Haggerty with Savoury Custard (see page 110)

MAKE-AHEAD MEAL FOR FRIENDS
- Labneh (see page 74)
- Mung Bean Humous with Sesame Pitta Crisps (see page 71)
- Freekeh, Herb and Black Olive Salad with Spiced Almonds (see page 138)
- Turnip, Olive and Preserved Lemon Tagine (see page 156)

SATURDAY IN-FRONT-OF-TV SUPPER
- Parmesan-crust Fries with Piri Piri Sauce (see page 181)
- Slow-rise Pan Pizza (see page 198)

CELEBRATORY SUMMER LUNCH
- Rösti Cups with Beet and Orange Relish (see page 184)
- Dolcelatte Tarts with Apple Nut Salad (see page 127)
- Fresh Summer Lasagne with Herb Oil (see page 212)

CELEBRATORY AUTUMN LUNCH
- Shallot Tarte Tatin (see page 150)
- Pear, Chestnut and Gorgonzola Winter Salad (see page 62)
- Porcini Risotto with Cavolo Nero and Cobnuts (see page 154)

INDIAN MEAL WITH FRIENDS
- Dosa with Coconut and Lime Chutney (see page 188)
- Chana Crispies with Mango Raita (see page 68)
- Kosheri (see page 52)
- Paneer Koftas in Spiced Yogurt Sauce (see page 189)

HALLOWE'EN GET-TOGETHER
- Sweetcorn Muffins with Avocado Salsa (see page 28)
- Corn Flatbread Pizzas (see page 84)
- Red Bean and Chocolate Chilli (see page 196)

SPECIAL SUMMER PICNIC
- Avocado Gazpacho (see page 56)
- Butternut Squash Scones with Goats' Cheese (see page 26)
- Sour Cherry, Red Quinoa and Spiced Almond Salad (see page 60)
- Hand-raised Mushroom Pie (see page 202)

Index

Acknowledgements

I've loved writing this book – it's been an interesting journey and I'd
like to think the finished result is all the better for it. I would really
like to thank the team at Watkins for staying with the book and for
all their support on this journey. As always, my heartfelt appreciation
goes to Grace Cheetham, for her ongoing support, belief and really
valued suggestions. I'd also like to thank designers Georgina Hewitt and
Allan Sommerville; and editors Wendy Hobson and Rebecca Woods
– it's been great to work with such talents. Huge thanks, too, to the
incredibly creative photographers, Liz and Max Haaralla Hamilton,
and food stylist Sara Lewis for making everything look so beautiful.